NATURAL SLEEP

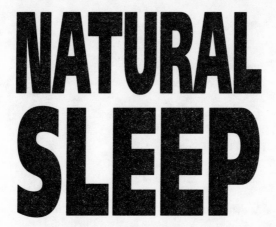

NATURAL SLEEP

How to Beat Insomnia Without Drugs

Anthea Courtenay

THORSONS PUBLISHING GROUP

First published 1990

British Library Cataloguing in Publication Data

Courtenay, Anthea
  Natural sleep: how to beat insomnia without drugs.
  1. Man. Insomnia. Self-treatment
  I. Title
  616.8498

ISBN 0 7225 1947 8

Published by Thorsons Publishers Limited, Wellingborough, Northamptonshire NN8 2RQ, England

Typeset by Harper Phototypesetters Limited, Northampton, England
Printed in Great Britain by Mackays of Chatham, Kent

10 9 8 7 6 5 4 3 2 1

Contents

Acknowledgements

I would like to thank the following people:
Chris Alford of the Sleep Laboratory, Leeds University
Brian Butler, director, The Association of Systematic Kinesiology
John Cape, clinical psychologist
Morag Chacksfield, medical herbalist
Bridgeen Doherty, reflexologist and aromatherapist
The Dulwich Health Centre, for information on geopathic stress
Tricia Donà-Hooker, aromatherapist
Christopher Eedy, osteopath and manipulative therapist
Dr Chris Hanning of the British Sleep Society
Dr Jim Horne, director, Sleep Laboratory, Loughborough University
Dr Julian Kenyon, director, The Centre for the Study of Complementary Medicine, Southampton
Maggie La Tourelle, kinesiologist and counsellor
Ron Lacey, director, MIND
William Lamble, homoeopath
Dr Christopher Mace, psychiatrist, St George's Hospital Sleep Clinic
Gloria May, hypnotherapist
Dr Margaret Macdonald, acupuncturist
Michael McIntyre, medical herbalist
Simon Mills, medical herbalist
Kate Morrison, naturopath and osteopath
Roger Newman Turner, acupuncturist, naturopath and osteopath
Delcia Thorpe, massage practitioner and subtle energy healer
Kathy Rees, for advice on anxiety
Jane Ware, clinical psychologist

Introduction

A good, uninterrupted night's sleep is one of the most enjoyable and totally natural pleasures available to us. Yet for many people it is hard to come by. It has been estimated that at some time half the British population will be affected by insomnia. According to a Harris Poll commissioned by the *Observer* (published in February 1990), 16 per cent of us suffer from insomnia, although it rises to as many as 21 per cent in Scotland and the North. Some sources place the number of adult insomniacs as high as 35 per cent at any one time.*

Insomnia not only causes stress; it is usually the result of stress. It is a sign that something in your life is out of balance: it may be emotional, environmental, or nutritional. It may be to do with your working life or lack of work, or to general unhappiness or depression. These are daytime problems, that need to be dealt with during the day.

Yet until recently the stock medical response has generally been to hand out a prescription for sleeping pills. In the Harris Poll, 12 per cent of those polled were taking sleeping pills, 9 per cent were taking tranquillizers and 7 per cent anti-depressants. In 1988 £15.9 million's worth of hypnotic drugs were prescribed, excluding those given directly by hospitals and doctors. This figure does *not* include the minor tranquillizers, which some people take to help them sleep.

GPs are becoming much less inclined to prescribe pills for insomnia; these days doctors as well as patients are concerned

*S.J.E. Lindsay and M. Jahanshi, 'Disorders of Sleep: Investigation', *A Handbook of Clinical Adult Psychology*, Stan Lindsay and Graham Powell (eds.), (Gower, 1987)

about the side-effects of drugs, in particular the long-term possibility of addiction. They know that drugs don't solve the problems underlying insomnia, but many of them lack the time and facilities to help patients deal with these.

A variety of natural, drugless treatments have been found successful in restoring sleep. Many forms of natural medicine, including homoeopathy, acupuncture, and herbalism can help sufferers to regain physical and emotional harmony. Both orthodox and complementary practitioners recognize the value of relaxation techniques, counselling, nutritional advice, or simply helping people to train themselves into new sleeping habits. Unfortunately most of these methods require expert time and attention, of which NHS workers only have limited supplies.

Despite the fact that insomnia is so widespread and can be treated, there are very few specialist facilities for its treatment in Britain. Only two or three sleep disorders clinics are available within the Health Service (there are also some in the private sector), and the number of sleep research laboratories is diminishing. And although the 1980s have seen the rise of self-help groups for all kinds of problems I have not, in researching this book, found one for non-sleepers. (If any exist, it would be useful to know about them!)

There are doctors, scientists and psychologists who would like to see more attention paid to the problem and more and better services made available. Towards the end of 1989 a number of experts from a wide range of disciplines, including sociology and neurophysiology as well as medicine and psychology, joined forces to set up the British Sleep Society. Its general aim is to promote the study and treatment of sleep disorders, and to inform GPs and other physicians about what services are available. (The Society, composed of very busy professionals, cannot offer a direct service to the public.)

Meanwhile, there is a great deal that most insomniacs can do for themselves. I am going to be looking at the different types of insomnia, their possible causes, how you can help yourself, and where to go for help if you need it. Take heart: according to psychologist and sleep researcher Dr Jacob Empson, 'the most intractable sleep disorders tend to be very rare'.*

*Jacob Empson, *Sleep and Dreaming*, (Faber & Faber, 1989)

You can change your sleeping patterns, if you really want to. But because the quality of your sleep usually reflects the quality of your daily life, you may have to be willing to make some other changes, too. And it is within the power of most of us to make changes in our attitudes and habits to bring about not only a better night's sleep but a happier daytime life.

PART 1

Sleep and insomnia

CHAPTER 1

What is sleep?

It is an extraordinary fact that something that occupies up to a third of our lives is still a mystery. Of course, we all know that sleep gives us rest: without it we feel tired and irritable and don't function as well as we'd like. Since 1952, sleep research laboratories attached to universities have been studying sleep patterns, with the help of human guinea-pigs. They have made numerous investigations not just into how we sleep but *why*, and no one has yet come up with a complete answer.

If you are beset by insomnia, you might wonder what use such investigations are. Whatever sleep is *for*, you know you need it and feel rotten without it. But the results of many of these investigations can offer some reassurance to the non-sleeper. They have, for instance, blown away the myth that everyone needs eight hours a night. Some of them suggest that most of us could get by on less sleep than we have without coming to harm. And some have come up with ideas for improving sleep.

During sleep all kinds of chemical and hormonal changes go on in our bodies; many of them are to do with bodily repair and restitution, and it has been thought that sleep was essential for these to occur. But at Loughborough University Dr Jim Horne, Director of the Sleep Research Laboratory, has come to a different conclusion. In his recent book *Why We Sleep* (Oxford University Press, 1988) he suggests that for most bodily repair processes sleep is not essential; they can take place just as well during periods of 'relaxed wakefulness'. Sleep, says Dr Horne, is needed mainly to rest the brain; this takes place during periods of very deep sleep, which he calls 'Core Sleep', occupying only part of our total night's sleep.

In sleep the brain goes through four main stages, each characterized by different types of brainwave — the electrical impulses emitted by the brain. In sleep laboratories these are measured by EEGs (electro-encephalograms), which are carried out by fixing electrodes to the sleeper's scalp with easily-removable glue. From these electrodes, amplified signals are recorded on paper by mechanical inkpens, or on magnetic tape, showing the activity of the cerebral cortex — the outer part of the brain. In the waking state our brains normally emit fast beta waves, which have a frequency of around 15 cycles per second. During the night, we go through several cycles of different brainwaves, each cycle lasting around 90 minutes.

Sleep states

Stage 1: This first stage, the lightest, is the transition from wakefulness to drowsiness; as we enter it our muscles relax, the blood pressure drops, and the heart rate and digestion slow down. The brain begins to produce hormones such as serotonin and melatonin which are associated with sleep and sleepiness (whether they actually *cause* sleep is under debate).

At the same time, there is an increase in alpha waves, brain-waves of 7-14 cycles per second, which are typical of relaxed wakefulness; alpha waves also appear in people who are medi-tating, or under hypnosis. This stage lasts between one and ten minutes in the normal sleeper; although we return to it at intervals during the night, it usually occupies only about 5 per cent of our sleep.

Stage 2: This stage starts quite soon after falling asleep and occupies about 45 per cent of human sleep. It contains a mixture of deeper, slower brainwaves: theta brainwaves (3.5-7.5 cycles per second) typical of drowsiness and light sleep, and slow delta waves (under 3.5 cycles per second), during which we are really unconscious.

Stage 3: which occupies only about 7 per cent of sleep in young adults, is another transition phase to deeper sleep; as delta wave activity increases, we are taken fairly rapidly into Stage 4.

Stage 4: is the deepest form of sleep, with delta brainwaves predominating; it makes up about 13 per cent of sleep in the young adult. We stay in Stage 4 for quite long periods before surfacing again to REM and Stage 1 several times during the night.

REM Sleep: Rapid Eye Movement sleep is so called because the sleeper's eyes move, indicating that they are dreaming. It occurs during Stage 1 sleep, and increases in quantity later on in the night. It has now been found that we also dream during deeper stages of sleep.

Core sleep

In *Why We Sleep* Dr Horne proposes that the really essential part of sleep consists of Stages 3 and 4, which he calls collectively Slow Wave Sleep (SWS). During these stages the brain is in what he calls on 'off-line' state: it is the only time during which this hard-working organ is totally at rest. SWS occurs largely during the first three cycles, that is, during the first half of a night's sleep.

When people are deprived of sleep by staying up all night, it has been found that they don't need to catch up with all the sleep they've lost. They recover no extra light sleep, and only a fraction of REM sleep. But they do recover all the lost deep sleep, which suggests that that is the sleep that is really essential.

In people who naturally need less sleep than the average, the same pattern is followed during the first few hours as in average sleepers. Although these people sleep for fewer hours, says Dr Horne, they are getting the essential Slow Wave Sleep: 'It is as though these short sleepers have somehow done away with what seems to be the flexible non-restorative sleep — the latter hours of sleep.'

His conclusion is that so long as we get our ration of Core Sleep, consisting of Slow Wave Sleep and some REM sleep, the brain will recover from its waking wear and tear. The rest he calls 'optional sleep', which has no essential purpose but 'fills the tedious hours of darkness until sunrise, maintaining sleep beyond the point where core sleep declines', and it may in fact not be really necessary.

How much sleep do we need?

The average young adult today sleeps for about seven and a half hours — but that's just an average. 65 per cent of you adults sleep between 6.5 and 8.5 hours, and 95 per cent between 5.5 and 9.5.

The amount of sleep needed, or taken, by individual people varies enormously. There's a standard belief that eight hours is the norm, but we all know of people who need much less. Mrs Thatcher is said to thrive on four or five, and there have been a number of other famous short sleepers, including Winston Churchill and Napoleon (both of whom catnapped during the day), Voltaire who only needed three hours, and Dostoyevsky, who wrote his books between 3 p.m. and 5 or 6 the next morning. I always envy short sleepers; think how much they can get done in those extra hours!

It's quite important for couples to realize that these variations are real; a short sleeper married to a long sleeper can make their partner's life quite difficult if they insist on banging around at six in the morning, or interpret the other's genuine needs as laziness.

Short and long sleepers have been found by and large to have different personalities. Short sleepers tend to be hard-working, ambitious, and rather obsessive, as well as extrovert and efficient. Long sleepers worry more, are less self-assured and value their sleep, which they may use as an escape. They are also often creative people — and creative people are said to dream more and to have more vivid and adventurous dreams than other people. Einstein was a long sleeper.

The amount of sleep taken by human beings has varied over the centuries. In 1910 a survey showed that young adults normally slept for nine hours a night, and before the advent of electricity most people adapted their sleep needs to the amount of daylight available, sleeping longer hours in winter, as Eskimos still do. I think a lot of us would do the same if working hours permitted; today's lifestyle, particularly in towns and cities, is not in keeping with natural rhythms, which is one very good reason why there are so many people with sleep problems today.

The ages of sleep

The amount of sleep we need also varies with age. The 'average' 7.5 applies to adults between 16 and 50. Most small babies sleep about 16-18 hours a day, and toddlers still need a lot more sleep than adults. However, some older children may actually need less than adults, something which parents don't always recognize. With adolescence, the picture changes; some teenagers will sleep up to 15 hours a night. They are not necessarily being lazy, and will grow out of it. However, parents should note that longer sleeping hours are also a symptom of depression, which can hit teenagers quite badly. At about the age of 16 we reach the 'normal' adult pattern — that is, whatever is normal for us.

From the age of 40 in men and 50 in women, the pattern alters again. In some women the menopause temporarily disrupts sleeping patterns. But in everyone, as they grow older, night-time sleep becomes lighter and more broken, with fewer dreams. In addition, many older people take naps during the day, so needing less sleep at night. Including catnaps, the average sleep for 70-year-olds is about six hours in 24. It's important to realize this, since many old people ask their doctors for help with their 'insomnia' when in fact they are sleeping quite normally for their age.

Within this overall pattern there are, as already mentioned, enormous variations. Some babies naturally need little sleep; some older people, especially if they remain active, don't catnap and retain a full night's sleep.

Your body clock: circadian rhythms

The functioning of our bodies is governed by a biological inner clock, known as the circadian rhythm (from the Latin *circa diem*, meaning 'about a day'). This regulates the times when various organs become more or less active, and when the production of various hormones peaks and tails off. The length of the circadian day is normally between 24 and 25 hours; some people have sleep problems because their body clocks are out of timing with the norm, or disturbed by things like shift work and jet lag.

The siesta, traditional in hot countries like Spain, is in decline as Mediterranean businesses come into line with the rest of

Europe. Yet it could be much more natural than our own patterns. The circadian rhythm is set to bring on sleep twice a day, mainly at night, but also in the early afternoon, which is why many people feel sleepy after lunch.

The circadian rhythm also varies with age. Babies sleep regularly during the day, at first at around three-hourly intervals, tailing off to a morning and an afternoon sleep; by the age of about two and a half they are sleeping in the afternoon only. In the elderly, the need for an afternoon sleep usually returns.

It appears to be the circadian rhythm which is responsible for some people being 'owls', finding it hard to wake in the morning but lively at night, while others are 'larks', leaping out of bed first thing and drooping by ten in the evening. Interestingly, these differences seem to grow less as people age.

REM Sleep — is your dreaming really necessary?

It used to be thought that the part of sleep essential to us was REM sleep, associated with dreaming; it was believed that these stages were needed for brain rest, and that people deprived of them would develop psychosis. This last has been disproved, though deprivation of REM sleep does produce irritability and difficulties in concentration, and affects the ability to retain information learned the day before. People totally deprived of it for more than three days have started having waking dreams, in the form of hallucinations. Others have been found to become less inhibited and conscientious!

In laboratories, REM sleep is measured by placing additional electrodes around the eyes to detect the eye movements, and over muscles in the chin or neck, which relax during sleep. During this time cells in the brain's cortex, the grey matter, are also electrically very active. REM sleep has also been called 'paradoxical sleep', because although the brain is active, the body experiences a kind of paralysis and can't move voluntarily; some people notice this when trying to awaken from a nightmare — it can be quite frightening.

Nearly all mammals dream; there are a few exceptions, like dolphins, who sleep with only one half of their brain at a time, presumably because they need to be aware of where they are in the ocean, and alert to predators. Humans dream about twice as much as most mammals, with a dreaming phase about every 90 minutes, though the amount of dreaming declines with age. New-born and even unborn babies spend an enormous amount of time in REM sleep, but whether they are actually dreaming can't be known for certain.

The average sleeper spends about an hour and a half a night in REM sleep, sometimes more; it starts about 45 minutes after falling asleep, and increases as the night goes on, with most dreaming taking place in the later part of the night, during 'optional' sleep.

Contrary to the belief that dreaming is essential for mental health, it has been found that depressed people, deprived of dreaming sleep by taking anti-depressant drugs for up to and over a year, actually felt better. Dr Horne suggests that dreams may not only be disturbing to a depressed person, but that too much dreaming may not be good for us.

However, for most people some REM sleep time does seem necessary, for when sleep laboratory subjects are deprived of these phases, there is a 'rebound effect': on recovery nights they take more REM sleep, making up about 50 per cent of what they have lost.

People have come up with all kinds of contradictory theories as to why we dream. The fathers of psychoanalysis, Freud and Jung, believed that dreams shed light on our hidden desires, and opened the way to the unconscious. Some contemporary research psychologists suggest that we dream to reorder stored information, and to consolidate memories and learning. Some researchers believe that dreams are the result of the brain discarding information, like wiping old computer programmes, and that remembering them is therefore actually bad for us. Dr Horne feels that REM sleep must have some importance, possibly as the 'cinema of the mind', a way of keeping the brain entertained during lighter stages of sleep.

What seems most likely is that all these theories are true: some dreams are simply junk-clearing; some simply result from indigestion. And some do serve as messengers from the unconscious, making you aware of unresolved problems, or suggesting solutions to them. People have certainly experienced dreams that are emotionally healing, or very creative. Both poetry and scientific ideas have been inspired by dreams — Robert Louis Stevenson is said to have dreamed the story of the best-selling *Dr Jekyll and Mr Hyde*. And there seems no doubt that a few dreams can be predictive.

If you are interested in dream content, it can be useful to keep a dream diary. As you note down your dreams every night, you may observe certain themes coming up regularly which could shed new light on your problems or your understanding of yourself. If you're not sure what a dream means, don't read books that give blanket meanings for dream symbols; by and large your dreams will choose symbols that are personally meaningful to you. Sometimes their meaning becomes clear in the process of writing them down.

As far as insomnia is concerned, dreams or nightmares are important when they are part of the problem, waking you up regularly or in a state of fear. If you have unpleasant recurring dreams, your unconscious mind may be trying to draw your attention to something that needs to be dealt with, perhaps a past traumatic event that you have not come to terms with, or a present problem like a difficult relationship. In such cases, some form of counselling, psychotherapy or hypnotherapy may help you unravel the message.

Meanwhile, states Dr Horne: 'Pleasant though dreams can be, it is possible that too much attention is paid to them and the importance of REM sleep. Evidence is growing that deep, non-dream sleep (Core Sleep) is more vital to well-being.'

CHAPTER 2

Insomnia

Insomnia is defined by sleep experts as difficulty in initiating and maintaining sleep, which has continued for at least three weeks. Chronic insomnia can last for years, while intermittent insomnia can be triggered by particular anxieties or crises. People experience insomnia in different ways: for some it's the tossing and turning for what feels like hours before they drop off; others wake up at intervals and feel they never get a good night; and others wake early in the morning, and can't get off to sleep again.

Insomnia can't be measured by the number of hours you sleep, since people's needs vary so much. It's been found in sleep laboratories that some insomniacs actually sleep longer than 'normal' sleepers: if you need ten hours and only sleep for eight, then you won't feel as refreshed as the good sleeper who needs seven.

Different types of insomnia have traditionally been related to different states of mind; it's often said that not being able to get off to sleep at night is a symptom of anxiety, while waking early is a sign of depression. Actually, it's not as simple as that. Some anxious and depressed people actually sleep more, presumably in an effort to escape from their feelings. Some depressed people can't get off to sleep, and some anxious people fall asleep normally, but wake in the small hours.

A number of sleep experts believe that anger and resentment are more frequent causes of insomnia than anxiety and depression. Others suggest that the over-active, churning mind may not be a cause of insomnia, but a result. In addition, there is often more than one factor involved; an over-active mind may be related to an under-active body, for example. And as you can see from the check-list below, the causes of sleeplessness are not always emotional.

Type of problem	Possible causes/ Contributory factors
Taking a long time to get to sleep (Most common in people under 30 and women)	Habit Emotional stress (anxiety, depression, unhappiness, anger, guilt etc) Unsolved problems Obsessive thinking Psychiatric disturbances Dietary factors: including too many junk foods, stimulating foods and drinks, and eating heavy meals late at night. Digestive problems Smoking, especially in the evenings Lack of regular exercise Stress (at home or work) Major life changes — moving house, divorce, changing jobs etc. Certain medical conditions Neurological problems Needing less sleep than you think you do Napping during the day Jet lag, working night shifts and other body clock disturbances External disturbances like noise

Type of problem	Possible causes/ Contributory factors
Waking during the night (more common in older people and men)	As above, plus: High degrees of anger and irritability Heavy alcohol consumption Withdrawal from alcohol or drugs (medical or otherwise) Nightmares Fear of nightmares (waking just before you are about to dream) Not being fully extended during the day
Waking early and not going back to sleep	As above, plus: Severe depression Sleeping pill dependency Alcoholism
Getting 'enough' sleep, but still feeling tired	Sleep apnea (see Part 2, Chapter 1) Pseudo-insomnia. (See below) Depression

Are you really insomniac?

True insomnia affects your daily life and performance. Even if you feel you don't sleep well, as long as you're not tired during the day, you're not insomniac. The real test is whether, as well as suffering from night-time wakefulness, you consistently feel sleepy, tired and irritable throughout the day, possibly affecting your memory, concentration and ability to work.*

However, *worrying* about your sleeplessness can be just as stressful as not sleeping. If you fall into any of the categories below, you may be worrying unnecessarily:

Ageing

Many elderly people find themselves waking in the early hours of the morning and misdiagnose themselves, or are misdiagnosed, as insomniac. Let's have a look at what's really happening.

As I've mentioned, as people grow older, most of them have more need to nap during the day. If your normal sleep ration is seven hours a night, and you have gradually added a couple of hours of daytime napping, those two hours cut into your ration of seven. If you then go to bed at ten, you will only need five hours' sleep, and will wake naturally at three in the morning, and — provided you don't worry about it — feel quite refreshed.

So, if you nap during the day, you have a choice: you can knock your snoozing time off your total required sleep time and accept less sleep in bed; if you wake early, get up or maybe read in bed. If you want to wake later, but start feeling sleepy between 9 and 10 p.m., have a half hour nap and go to bed later. Whichever you choose to do, enjoy it, and stop worrying.

It is also normal for older people to sleep more lightly than they once did, with more frequent wakenings. Everyone has very brief moments of waking or near-waking as they come out of the REM cycles during the night, but we don't usually remember them. As you get older those moments may turn into minutes; if you start worrying about it, that in itself will keep you awake. If you realize that there's nothing wrong with you, you can enjoy the sensation of being awake but resting, cosily wrapped up in

---

*Daytime sleepiness can be a symptom of other sleep disorders than insomnia, including the respiratory problem sleep apnea (see Part 2, Chapter 1), sufferers from which may not be aware that they are losing sleep. Narcolepsy also produces daytime sleepiness: the sufferer sleeps normally but also drops off at inopportune moments during the day. It is a rare condition, for which there are drug treatments; it can also be treated with homoeopathy. Sufferers can help themselves to some extent by avoiding foods high in carbohydrates.

the warm. Only start worrying if the minutes really turn into hours, if you feel too miserable to enjoy them, or if you are missing out on total sleep time, taking naps into account.

The fact that a changing sleep pattern is normal as we age doesn't mean that the eldery don't ever suffer from insomnia, perhaps compounded by a medical condition. It's too easy to dismiss problems as 'just your age'. If you take the advice above, and are still not getting the sleep you need, and are perhaps feeling depressed and run down as well, do please read the rest of this book.

You don't need as much sleep as you think

Some people are brought up on the idea that eight hours is essential, when they perhaps only need five. Convinced they haven't had enough sleep, they may lie in in the mornings to catch up, which simply compounds the problem.

If you take a long time getting off to sleep and are not suffering from any other kind of stress or anxiety, nor particularly tired, start getting up very regularly at the same time; don't have lie-ins or naps. Then go to bed half an hour later each night, until you find yourself falling asleep within a few minutes. After that, go to bed when you feel sleepy, and not before.

Faulty body clocks

A few people seem to have a biological fault in their circadian rhythm, which can be detected in a sleep disorders clinic. At the Sleep-Wake Disorders Center at Montefiore Hospital in New York, the late Dr Elliot Weitzman found that a number of patients had a chronic inability to fall asleep until around 4-5 a.m., when they slept quite well. However, as they had to get up to go work, they were always short of sleep. They didn't respond to sleeping pills, and they didn't seem to be suffering from any other sort of stress. There was apparently a fault in the mechanism regulating the time of sleep onset.

The solution found was for these people to go to bed three hours later every night, when they slept for eight hours, for six days running, so that their day was lengthened to 27 hours during this period. This finally brought them round to a bedtime of 11 p.m., by which time their clocks seemed to have been reset, since the majority of them continued to go to bed at 11 p.m.

A pattern of late-sleeping and late-waking can develop among young people and students as a result of their lifestyle — staying up late studying or partying and then catching up in the mornings can develop into a habit. The only way to break it is to be very firm with yourself about getting up regularly at the same, earlier time.

A very few people have body clocks that are really out of sync with the rest of the world. One young woman could never get to sleep when the rest of the world did; it was found that she had a circadian day of 36-38 hours. Once she had understood the cause of her problem, she made the most of it. She became a freelance writer, working for 20-22 hours a day, and then relaxing for some hours before going to bed and sleeping for 10-12 hours.*

Pseudo-insomnia

This rather rude label doesn't mean you are malingering. Objectively, sufferers fall asleep within 20 minutes and get at least six hours' sleep; but they complain they 'haven't slept a wink'. It seems that the quality of their sleep is not sufficiently deep for them to feel refreshed. Most normal sleepers change positions 30-40 times and wake four or five times each night, but so briefly that they don't remember waking; lighter sleepers who are aware of these waking moments can feel that they have tossed and turned all night. When the brainwaves of pseudo-insomniacs are monitored in sleep laboratories, some of them appear to be thinking all night while asleep; some actually spend the night dreaming that they are awake. One suggested explanation is that their body functions remain active after they have fallen asleep, giving them the feeling of being awake.

In her book *Sleep Like a Dream* (Sheldon Press, 1988), Rosemary Nicol suggests making a note of the time every ten minutes throughout the night, mentally or on a slip of paper. If you miss noting a ten-minute stage, you have been sleeping. Knowing this may help you to worry less and sleep better. So will paying attention to a balanced lifestyle and learning to relax.

*Peter Hauri, Ph.D, *The Sleep Disorders* (Upjohn, 1977)

Shift work

This is an artificial cause of body clock disturbance. Most people who have to go to bed in the morning and sleep till mid-afternoon take a week or ten days to adapt to the new pattern. It's not just their sleep that has to adapt, but the whole circadian rhythm involving the timing of hormone release and other bodily functions. Problems arise when working hours are regularly changed, or when the shift worker tries to return to a normal pattern on a day or weekend off. If you have to work at nights, remember that your body clock needs at least a week to adjust to a new schedule.

You are worrying unduly about falling asleep

Most people take 10-20 minutes to get to sleep. In one sleep laboratory study, a self-styled insomniac complained that he took hours to fall asleep. However, his brainwave patterns showed that he fell asleep within 20 minutes, just like any normal sleeper; his concern about his 'insomnia' made the 20 minutes feel like hours.

Quality versus quantity

Insomnia is unpleasant. It is boring and uncomfortable in itself, and it can affect your daily activities, work and relationships. However, it may not be quite as damaging as some insomniacs fear. Sleep research laboratories have shown that people who normally sleep for seven to eight hours can adapt over time to as much as two hours' less sleep daily without impairing their mental or physical ability. And when people have been totally deprived of sleep for between eight and eleven days (the longest times so far studied) most of the body's organs, except for the brain, continue to function remarkably well. While the brain does need rest, Dr Horne stresses that 'everything else from the neck down seems to cope very well, without sleep, provided you get regular rest and regular food.'

Nevertheless, too little sleep can and does affect us, both because of genuine fatigue, but also because we *believe* that shortened sleep will cause us suffering. Our beliefs about how things should be have a major effect on how we react to them.

So, how much sleep do we really need?

Dr Horne believes that around six hours is more than adequate for mental health; any sleep after that comes into his category of 'optional sleep'. If his theory is correct, what the brain needs is Core Sleep, the deep slow-wave sleep. This should provide some reassurance to insomniacs: Core Sleep predominates during the first sleep cycles, so even if you only sleep for a few hours, you will be getting a period of this important deep sleep, together with some REM sleep.

Conditions in sleep laboratories, of course, where the human guinea-pigs are fed and rested, and have chosen to lose sleep, are quite different from those of the person tossing and turning in the lonely small hours — even if they end up getting the same amount of sleep, which is possible. EEG readings show that most insomniacs actually sleep much more than they claim to: quite often people who feel they have only slept an hour or two have actually slept for several. It appears that people's *perception* of their insomnia can cause as much stress as the insomnia itself, and it may well be that *worrying* about insomnia can make you just as stressed, tetchy and tired as not sleeping. It will also contribute to keeping you awake.

So, if you are insomniac, there are three important things to remember. Firstly, you may be getting more sleep than you think. Secondly, so long as you get some sleep and can relax your body, you will not come to long-term harm. Thirdly, your attitude towards your sleep has a lot to do with the quality of the sleep you get.

The first step towards beating insomnia is not to worry about it.

PART 2

Dealing with the cause

CHAPTER 1

Seeking the cause

As we've seen, there are many possible causes of insomnia. If you were referred to a sleep disorders clinic, you would be taken through a detailed questionnaire covering your medical history and general health, state of mind, relationships, past history, eating and drinking habits, and recent life, as well as your actual sleep patterns.

Your sleeping arrangements are also important; you'd be asked where you sleep, who with, and about your relationship with that person. (Your sleeping partner, if you have one, would probably be invited along as well.) In this way a very complete picture would be built up, in order to disentangle what's causing or contributing to your insomnia.

Sometimes quite simple answers are rapidly found — too much coffee-drinking for example. Sometimes the reasons are more worrying, like alcoholism or drug addiction. Very often the causes relate to emotional stress, including worry about the insomnia itself.

In certain cases, you might be asked to spend a couple of nights in a sleep laboratory. You'd spend one night acclimatizing, and on the second you'd be wired up to have your brain-waves charted during the night. Through computer analysis a hypnogram would be produced, a summary diagram of your sleep pattern, showing how much of the night you spend in sleep and how much awake, when you are awake and for how long, and also the quality of your sleep. It would show how much time you were spending in deep slow-wave sleep, transitional sleep, and REM sleep. Without sufficient slow-wave sleep you might not feel completely rested; while if you were short on REM sleep you might also feel mentally tired.

In a sleep clinic, once a detailed assessment has been made, a strategy would be worked out with you for improving your sleep. In this book you can be your own sleep clinician, asking yourself what applies to you, and what you can do about it. And probably the first thing a sleep expert would do would be to ensure that you've had a thorough medical check-up.

Getting a check-up

Although insomnia is most commonly related to emotional stress, sometimes the causes can be partly or even totally physical or environmental. Mind and body are interdependent: our brains and nervous systems, for instance, are affected by chemical factors including food and pollution, both of which can trigger mental stress. This in turn leads to physical depletion and possibly illness, which creates further stress.

But since there are some specific medical problems associated with sleep disorders, it may be sensible — if you haven't already done so — to have a check-up with your doctor or a well-qualified alternative practitioner. Some of the natural therapies described in Part 4 can be very helpful in treating or relieving the problems asterisked below.*

These are some of the conditions a practitioner might look out for:

Alcoholism

People who regularly drink large amounts of alcohol tend to wake early, after a lighter sleep than the norm, while chronic alcoholics show the sleep pattern of the aged, with many awakenings, little or no delta sleep, and decreased REM sleep, but extra sleepiness during the day.

*Allergies

Allergies to food, drink, and chemicals in food, water, the atmosphere and furnishings, can give rise to many of the mood disturbances associated with insomnia like depression, anxiety, and nervousness, as well as physical symptoms. Some allergies also cause daytime sleepiness. (See the section on Allergies and Sensitivities, in Part 3, Chapter 3.)

*Anorexia nervosa

These patients tend to sleep little and wake up frequently during the night. When anorexics start returning to normal eating patterns and put on some weight, their sleep also begins to normalize.

Apnea

This is a fairly recently recognized problem. Sufferers may be less aware of it than their sleeping partners, for the sign of apnea is loud, irregular snoring. Between 1 and 4 per cent of the population may be affected, mostly male.

Sleep apnea occurs in people who have an obstruction at the back of the throat; as the throat relaxes in sleep, their breathing is cut off and the oxygen level in the blood drops. They don't usually awake fully, but reach a near waking state in order to breathe again, usually with a loud snort, sometimes accompanied by thrashing around. In severe cases this can happen every few minutes throughout the night. As a result, apnea sufferers never get into the deep stage of sleep, and are tired throughout the day. They can suffer from loss of concentration and memory, and are at risk of nodding off at meetings, or while driving. Apnea can also strain the heart. The danger is that these symptoms can be confused with 'getting older'.

The majority of sufferers are male, often overweight and heavy drinkers. Being overweight makes the condition worse by narrowing the throat further, and alcohol, particularly late at night, relaxes the throat muscles, as do sleeping pills.

So if your partner has a distinct snoring pattern, regularly stopping for 20-30 seconds and starting again with a loud snort, and if he or she also complains of daytime tiredness, do persuade him or her to get medical advice.

The first steps towards recovery are to lose weight and cut down on alcohol, particularly at night. Treatments include surgery, or wearing a mask attached to a pump which blows air into the throat to stop the muscles from collapsing downward.

In children apnea may be caused by enlarged tonsils, or a structural abnormality in the jaw. They may grow out of it, but if it is affecting their daytime behaviour, do get an expert opinion.

Caffeine addiction

This is a widespread cause of sleeplessness; a GP tells me that most of his 'insomniac' patients turn out to be coffee freaks. Caffeine is not only contained in coffee, but in tea, chocolate and cola drinks; it is a drug on which many people develop a dependency. Although it is a well known stimulant, some people drink ten or twenty cups of coffee or tea every day, and wonder why they can't sleep at night. Even if you don't drink it in the evening, taking a lot during the day can disrupt sleep; the body can only process so much at once, and caffeine can remain in the system for several hours after consumption.

Not everyone is sensitive to coffee, but it's worth noting that when normal sleepers in a sleep laboratory at Leeds University were given coffee late at night, it not only delayed sleep onset by around 40 minutes but also affected the subjects' quality of sleep and performance next day. The sure-fire way to find out whether caffeine is causing or contributing to your insomnia is to stop drinking coffee and tea for a few days.

*Environmental factors

Environmental factors, such as geopathic stress, are recognized by only a few doctors, but can have an important effect on your health, mood and sleep. This subject is dealt with more fully in Part 2, Chapter 8.

*Heavy metal poisoning

Metal poisoning, for example from mercury, aluminium, and lead can also affect the system and keep you awake. Its presence can be tested by hair and blood analysis from a good allergy testing clinic. Nutritional advice, together with supplements including Vitamin C, garlic and kelp, can help to clear your system.

*Hyper-thyroidism

This is caused by an over-active thyroid gland which causes weight loss, shaky hands, anxiety, and fragmented, short sleep.

*Iatrogenic problems

These are induced by medical drugs, including sleeping pills which can prevent normal sleep. (See below.) Some individuals react badly to medical drugs which don't affect others; if the cause of your insomnia is a mystery, ask yourself whether it started around the time when you began taking a new form of medication.

*The menopause

This can affect some women's sleeping patterns as hormones adjust themselves to major change, often causing broken sleep. Night sweats can be an additional and annoying cause of sleep disturbance. Sleep usually settles down once the menopause is over, though owing to the ageing process it may be lighter than before.

For some women, the menopause brings home the realities of ageing, children leaving home, and so on, creating further depression and anxiety. A positive approach to this new, challenging phase of life can make a great difference to the severity of symptoms. A possible treatment for menopausal symptoms generally is HRT (Hormone Replacement Therapy), but views on its long-term safety differ both among doctors and natural therapists.

*Pain

Pain can be very disruptive to sleep; it often seems worse at night, and chronic pain is very depressing. If you know the cause and have been told nothing can be done, have you explored all possible medical avenues, such as getting referred to your local Pain Relief Clinic, or to a physiotherapist?

If you've been told you have to 'live with it', it may still be worth seeing an alternative practitioner; natural therapies can often relieve symptoms, even when they cannot guarantee a cure. Your approach to pain is important too. You can do a lot for yourself through relaxation, meditation, and your mental attitude. (See the section on Relaxation and Meditation in Part 3, Chapter 2.)

*Restless legs

This is an absolutely infuriating syndrome consisting of discomfort in one or both legs, and the urge to keep moving them; it keeps you awake even when the rest of you wants to sleep. Its cause is something of a mystery, but it may be connected with poor circulation, and/or lack of calcium or other nutrients including Vitamin E. In women it may be related to hormone levels. It is often worse when the sufferer is under stress.

One tactic is to improve the circulation in your legs by taking a footbath in alternate hot and cold water during the evening. Calcium in the form of Dolomite tablets taken at bedtime can be helpful.

Sudden weight loss

A sudden loss of weight through dieting can temporarily disrupt sleeping patterns.

Formulating a strategy

In a sleep clinic, once a detailed assessment has been made, a strategy would be worked out with you for improving your sleep. If you were found to be severely depressed, drug therapy might be recommended for a time. And of course if you were found to be suffering from a medical, neurological or psychiatric illness, you would be referred for appropriate treatment.

For most people, the options could include relaxation training, or a behavioural programme to restructure your sleeping habits. Or you might be referred to a psychiatrist or a clinical psychologist to help you deal with emotional stress. Psychological help might take the practical form of helping you to deal with anxiety by sorting out your priorities. You might be considered a suitable candidate for cognitive therapy, a way of learning how to change negative and anxious thoughts and beliefs about yourself. You might be helped by hypnotherapy, which a few psychiatrists and psychologists practise; or it might be considered that you would benefit from psychotherapy. We'll be looking at these options in the next few chapters.

Sleeping pills (a last resort)

Publicity about the side-effects of sleeping pills and tranquillizers belonging to the benzodiazepine group of drugs has made the general public wary of taking them, and doctors wary of prescribing them. When they were first produced in the 1960s they seemed to answer all sorts of problems: now we know that these drugs don't solve any problems, and can be extremely addictive.

In addition, when taken as sleeping pills, benzodiazepines reduce the quality of your sleep. They cause suppression of REM sleep in the first part of the night, often with a rebound effect with more dreaming later in the night, which can cause early wakening. They can also leave people feeling fuzzy-minded next morning, which is particularly dangerous in the old, since it can make them confused and increases the risk of falls.

Recently some new sleeping pills have come on the market, the cyclopirolones, which don't disturb normal sleep patterns. They haven't been around long enough for their long-term effects to be known for certain, and it's likely that doctors would discourage patients from taking them consistently for any length of time.

There may be a case for taking medication for a day or two under certain conditions — after the shock of a bereavement, for instance. But no one should take sleeping pills for year after year, as has been the case in the past.

What if you are already taking them? There have been many stories about the horrors of withdrawal symptoms. That may make you scared of giving them up, even if publicity about their effects on your sleep is also causing you anxiety.

1. Not everyone goes through horrendous withdrawal symptoms; a less well publicized fact is that numbers of people have given up sleeping pills relatively easily. Since we all have individual body and brain chemistry, the effects of both taking and giving up benzodiazepines can vary a great deal.

2. Giving them up is really worth it. Once they are out of your system you will return to a normal, natural sleep pattern, and your mind will be clearer.

3. It's vital to come off them slowly, by gradually tapering off

the dosage over at least two or three months; the worst with-drawals happen when people give them up suddenly. Some people try reducing their intake by cutting their pills in halves or quarters, but this method is not very accurate. It's best to consult your doctor so that he or she can prescribe gradually smaller doses. Your GP may be able to refer you to other sources of help, too, such as a relaxation class or self-help group. Some GPs are in touch with natural therapists and may be able to suggest someone reliable who can help you, through massage, aromatherapy, or hypnotherapy, for example.

Practitioners of natural therapies can be very supportive in helping you to come off sleeping pills, or dealing with the after-effects of coming off. They are not allowed to recommend you to go against your doctor's advice; you can of course make your own decision, but it's best if you work in co-operation with your doctor. Some natural practitioners prefer people to give up sleeping pills before starting treatment, either because the drugs may interfere with their treatment, or because they like to know that the patient is committed to stopping.

A hypnotherapist was asked to treat a woman with agora-phobia, who had already been helped by a herbalist to wean herself off the tranquillizers and anti-depressants she had taken for eight years. On her first visit, the woman's husband came with her because she couldn't go out alone; on her second, she came by herself. The hypnotherapist commented: 'She was very, very committed to her own recovery. She was going to do it! That commitment is something the therapist can't supply.'

What natural practitioners can supply is the time and the listening ear that busy GPs are rarely able to give, together with natural treatments to strengthen and detoxify the body. A naturopath and osteopath tells me that about 5 per cent of her patients are hooked on sleeping pills when they come to her. They usually come for treatment for some other problem, and after a while ask for her help in giving up the pills. She has found it possible to help them by using herbal pills as a bridge, and combining counselling with her physical treatments.

On giving up benzodiazepines, some people experience increased fatigue for a time, and some increased agitation. There can also be a period of increased dreaming. And it can happen that the suppressed anxieties for which they originally took the pills start surfacing. This is easier to cope with if you accept it as part of the healing process rather than a sign of sickness: it shows that these feelings are now on their way out. Counselling from a professional counsellor or alternative practitioner can help you through this stage.

Herbal sedatives

Practitioners of natural therapies would much rather help you to solve your sleeping problems altogether than be dependent on medication, but herbal tranquillizers can be useful and safe as a temporary prop while you recover your normal sleep.

Over 90 sedative herbal pills can currently be bought over the counter at health food shops and some chemists. Most of them contain slightly differing proportions of the same ingredients including valerian, scullcap, passiflora, wild lettuce and other sleep-inducing herbs. They can be taken during the day to counteract anxiety as well as to help you sleep at night.

Most herbal remedies are very mild, without the mind-deadening effect that chemical tranquillizers can induce, and they are not technically addictive; however it is possible to become psychologically dependent on them. While preferable to chemical drugs, there is still a risk of using them as a substitute for really dealing with your insomnia, and taken regularly for a few weeks on the trot their effectiveness can be reduced.

Herbal pills in general have no side-effects, and are safe to take; their sale is supervised by the Committee of Safety on Medicines. In 1989 newspapers reported that a woman had suffered liver damage after regularly taking a herbal tranquillizer; however, after investigation, the pills were not withdrawn from the market. Sometimes a herbal remedy is blamed when the person taking it has also been taking medication which could cause liver damage. Very occasionally, a person has an individual allergic reaction to a herbal product, which does not mean that it is dangerous to the rest of the population.

It says much for the safety of herbal pills that one case of a bad reaction can make the headlines, in comparison with the thousands of people suffering from tranquillizer addiction, and the hundreds who die every year from an accidental overdose of paracetamol-based drugs.

Buying herbal remedies

Among the numerous herbal sedatives on sale, some of the practitioners I have spoken to recommend Quiet Life, Neurelax, Passiflora, Kalms and Weleda's Avena sativa comp. Your health food store manager should also be able to give you some guidance.

Arkopharma products, made in France and available at good health stores, are very pure products containing single herbs for a variety of ailments. For insomnia there is a choice of four relating to different combinations of symptoms. One of their advantages is that purchasers can contact medical herbalists for free telephone advice.

For further information about herbal remedies, see the sections on Bedtime Drinks in Part 3, Chapter 4, and on Medical Herbalism in Part 4.

CHAPTER 2

The habit of insomnia

Whatever the cause or causes of your insomnia, sleeplessness is nearly always a symptom of some kind of disharmony in your daytime life. This disharmony may be mental, emotional, physical or environmental, often a combination. But whatever it is, it needs to be faced and dealt with during the day. By the time you get to bed, it's really too late.

Poor sleep can be exacerbated by bad eating and drinking habits, lack of exercise, and other physical and environmental factors which contribute further to tension and stress. We'll be looking at all of these in due course. But since your physical habits usually reflect your view of yourself, let's look first at the mental and emotional side.

The most important thing is to realize that you *can* do something. To decide what to do, you will need to look at your attitudes and lifestyle and possibly ask yourself a few questions. But once you start on a plan of action you will not only improve your sleep pattern but start creating for yourself a happier, more satisfying daytime life. As you read on, note what applies to you, and what you personally can change.

Sleep and habit

If your insomnia has become severe enough or prolonged enough for you to be reading this book, then it is in part a habit, perhaps alongside some other habits, like not looking after yourself well enough, or postponing dealing with anxieties. And short-term insomnia can become long-term insomnia simply by acquiring the habit of expecting to sleep badly.

Human beings are odd creatures: most of us like to think we

are independent, free-thinking spirits. Yet a surprising amount of our behaviour is totally conditioned, starting when we are very young. Much of our conditioning is helpful and life-supporting; it would be very inconvenient if every time you crossed a road you had to relearn the desirability of looking both ways, or what red, amber and green lights mean. Unfortunately the mechanical part of our brain absorbs other, less helpful lessons, like associating bed with lying awake.

It's common these days for the brain to be likened to a computer — a computer more vast and complex than any yet built, and of course with a capacity for original thought, but nonetheless a machine which obediently reproduces whatever programming is fed into it.

Thus a few people are 'sleep hypochondriacs'; early in life an over-anxious parent has programmed them with the idea that without eight hours' solid sleep their health will suffer. The computer part of the brain that has accepted this belief reacts with anxiety when those solid eight hours aren't forthcoming — until the owner of the computer takes a fresh look at the old programme and decides to delete it and feed in new, up-to-date information.

Of course, we are *more* than our brains, and our brains are much more than computers; but the image is useful in that a computer is amenable to instruction by the person in charge — you. The mechanical part of our thinking is intended as a tool, not a hindrance, and you have the power to change your unwanted programmes for more useful ones.

If your insomnia has an emotional basis, you may need to deal with that too. Meanwhile, how you think and talk to yourself may be creating a habit out of what could be a temporary problem.

Self-talk

The best way to break unhelpful habits is to start exchanging them for helpful ones. The first thing is to recognize in what particular ways your habitual thinking or behaviour is keeping you in that sleepless groove. How do you talk to yourself and others about your sleep? If you label yourself 'insomniac' and tell yourself every time you head for bed that it'll take you ages to get to sleep, you are simply reinforcing the programming that keeps you awake. You can change some of that thinking now, by telling yourself that you are now on the way to improving your sleep, and by no longer telling other people that you suffer from insomnia.

Be honest with yourself about this. Lots of people 'enjoy' their ailments. In some cases this can be an excuse for avoiding things they don't want to do, or even living a more fulfilled life. I would stress that this kind of pattern is very rarely deliberate: it's often another conditioned response, perhaps going back to a time when being ill got a child more of its mother's love and attention than when he or she was well. Never sleeping well may prevent people like this from facing up to other problems, or taking on new ventures which would mean change. That doesn't mean they are purposefully choosing not to sleep, but it's possible that lack of sleep has secondary advantages, like making their families feel sorry for them.

Could this apply to you? And if it does, do you really want to be someone others feel sorry for? Close your eyes and imagine for a moment telling your spouse or workmates, 'I slept wonderfully last night!' How does it feel? Probably uncomfortable at this moment, because it isn't true. How comfortable would it feel if it were true?

Start noticing your habitual thoughts about insomnia. In particular, look out for sentences beginning 'I always . . .' or 'I never . . .' or 'I know . . .' For example:

'*I always take hours to get to sleep*' or '*I always wake up for hours in the middle of the night.*'

These statements may not actually be true, although they feel true to you. As we've seen, most insomniacs over-estimate how long they take to get to sleep or lie awake during the night. You could make a start by recognizing that your perception of the amount of sleep you get may be inaccurate.

'*I'm never going to get to sleep tonight*' is another habitual statement which is an excellent way of programming your brain to stay awake.

'*I know I'll feel dreadful if I can't get to sleep.*' Of course, lack of sleep makes you tired, but you can also talk yourself into feeling worse. There are alternatives, such as telling yourself that even though you'd like more sleep, your body is still getting all the rest it needs.

Make a game of catching these kinds of thoughts. It may help you to write them down. Then try replacing your negative statements with positive ones; a good start might be: 'I'm now learning how to sleep better.' Make your positive statements ones you can believe. Telling yourself 'I am going to sleep perfectly tonight' may not work, because at this point you probably won't believe it, and trying to convince yourself will set up further tension. But you could try: 'I will take tonight as it comes.' You may be surprised by the results.

Starting to change your self-talk can be a way of opening up other possibilities. Once you realize that you don't have to be a victim of your own thinking and reactions, all kinds of barriers can begin to crumble.

Conditioned insomnia

A very few cases of insomnia are purely habitual, but they are interesting, because they show how strong conditioning can be. Insomnia often starts with a short-term crisis or emotional upset; for most people, normal sleep returns once the crisis is over. But for others, not sleeping becomes a habit which can last a very long time.

One woman suffered from insomnia for 20 years, which began when she had a nervous breakdown. She had long since recovered from the breakdown and the reasons for it; she had simply developed, at a time when she was vulnerable, the habit of not sleeping. She visited a hypnotherapist for a totally unrelated problem; on her third session she fell spontaneously into a very deep sleep. The therapist wrapped her in a rug and left her for an hour before waking her. When she got home she slept for the rest of the day and through the night. The pattern was broken, and she returned to normal sleep.

Insomnia quite often starts during an emotional crisis, when the sufferer's pre-bed routine, the bedroom and even the bed, become associated with unhappiness and sleeplessness. People whose insomnia is conditioned in this way often sleep very well in strange beds when they go away — or in even odder circumstances.

A 19-year-old American student usually took two to three hours to fall asleep. As a child he had lain awake, anxious and unhappy, listening to his parents' violent quarrels. They were divorced when he was 13, but his insomnia continued. He had two years of psychotherapy, but although his therapist found him remarkably healthy in view of his family difficulties, his sleep didn't improve. Asked to describe his best night's sleep during the past year, he said that it had been during a mountain-climbing expedition; forced by circumstances to spend the night on a cold, narrow ledge, tied to the rocks, he fell asleep almost immediately and had a very good night! In those desperately uncomfortable surroundings there were no associations with his childhood anxiety.*

Much conditioned insomnia starts in childhood. People who were sent to bed when they were small for being naughty may subconsciously associate bed and bedtime with anger and punishment. Some children are sent to bed for adult convenience long before they are really sleepy; they lie awake feeling bored and frustrated, developing a habit of wakefulness which continues into adulthood.

These negative feelings are enhanced if the child overhears family rows, or even their parents entertaining friends and having a good time. The children of single parents can feel particularly excluded if they are suddenly packed off to bed when a friend or lover arrives. Lying in bed becomes associated with anxiety, or a feeling of being unwanted, feelings which can also spill over into everyday life. You can begin to make changes to ensure that bedtime and your bedroom become associated with sleep, not sorrow.

Changing the pattern

A popular way of treating insomnia today is a behavioural psychology method called stimulus-control, which consists of retraining yourself to sleep by learning to associate bed and bedtime with sleep, and sleep alone. This is the routine:

1. Use your bed and bedroom for sleep only. Don't watch television, listen to the radio, read, work, smoke or eat in bed. Making love is of course permitted!

*Peter Hauri, Ph.D, *The Sleep Disorders*, (Upjohn, 1977)

2. Always get up at the same time, including weekends and holidays. Lie-ins may be tempting, but if you take more sleep than you need on Sunday morning it'll be harder to get to sleep on Sunday night.

If you find waking up really difficult, place your alarm clock at the other side of the room so that you have to get up to turn it off. Put the light on straight away, as light can stimulate wakefulness.

3. Don't take naps during the day. You can overcome post-lunch sleepiness with some deep breathing, or a quick walk round the block.

4. Don't go to bed until you are really sleepy.

5. If you don't fall asleep within ten minutes, get up and do something else *in another room*. Don't go back to bed until you are ready to fall asleep. The same applies if you wake up in the middle of the night for any length of time. Don't associate your bedroom with lying awake. Get up, make yourself a hot drink if you like — milk or herbal tea, but not coffee or ordinary tea. Read, or write letters, until you are ready to go to sleep again. (Some people do quite a lot of creative work in the middle of the night and don't miss their sleep at all.)

This method doesn't necessarily suit everybody, but some studies show that it can be successful. In one trial a group of elderly insomniacs with an average age of 67 were able to reduce their time for falling asleep from an average of over an hour to half an hour.[*]

There are further sleep-assisting habits you can develop:

1. Deal with specific anxieties during the day or early evening.

2. Avoid stimulating foods and drinks in the evening. These include coffee, tea and alcohol. Smoking is also a stimulant; if you can't give it up immediately, at least cut down, especially in the evening.

3. Avoid stimulating activities late at night, including strenuous exercise, work, and arguments.

[*]S.J.E. Lindsay and M. Jahanshi, 'Disorders of Sleep: Investigation', *A Handbook of Clinical Psychology*, Stan Lindsay and Graham Powell (eds.), (Gower, 1987)

4. Establish a winding-down routine before you go to bed. Spend the last hour before bedtime preparing for sleep, including some relaxation and a warm bath. (There's more about winding-down in Part 3.)

5. Make sure your bedroom is both well-aired and warm.

A word about naps

For good sleepers, daytime naps can be beneficial and restorative; as we've seen, the human body clock actually seems built for sleep twice a day. However, while you are recovering a normal sleep pattern, naps are best avoided. The exception here would be parents of new babies, who are not technically insomniac, but are getting broken nights. If you are elderly and the need for a daytime nap becomes overpowering, take it but remember to allow for less sleep at night.

CHAPTER 3

Restoring the balance

Our brains aren't purely computers. The human brain is divided in two, like a walnut, and each half has specific functions. As a rule the left hemisphere controls the right side of the body, and deals with functions like speech and logical thinking. The right hemisphere, controlling the left side of the body, is responsible for abstract thought, dreaming, intuition, and visual imagery. In a few people, the sides are reversed.

To be in harmony with ourselves, both sides of the brain need to be equally active, and to work in co-operation with each other. In this hectic world most people use the logical side most of the time, at the expense of the intuitive, imaginative side. To restore the balance, the day-dreaming part of our minds needs to be exercised as much as the logical part.

A left-right imbalance is often reflected in the physical body; people can be quite lop-sided without realizing it, because they are putting all their energies into one aspect of themselves. Alternative therapies like osteopathy, kinesiology and the Alexander Technique can help to correct this.

The intuitive hemisphere has been called the gateway to the unconscious; through it we can get in touch with our creativity and inspiration, our hidden desires, needs, memories, and inner wisdom. It is this side of the brain that comes up with brilliant flashes of intuition, or solutions to problems that logic has been unable to solve. Have you ever found that when you stop worrying about a problem and let it go, the answer just pops in — sometimes during a dream, sometimes when you wake up in the morning? Quietening the chatter of the logical brain gives the creative side a chance to help us.

Yet we have been taught to neglect it. You could compare the two hemispheres to a hard-working, serious-minded parent, and a creative child who wants to play. The parent concentrates on telling the child how to behave, and doesn't listen to what it has to say. Yet given a chance, the creative child can come up with original ideas and solutions that the conformist parent hasn't considered.

When mind and body are allowed to relax, the activity of the two hemispheres starts to equalize. At the same time, the brain-waves slow down from the active, busy beta rate, producing the alpha-rhythm that normally precedes sleep. We become both more peaceful and more creative.

This state of mind can be achieved in a number of ways, for instance through relaxation and meditation (which I'll be returning to in Part 3), and through the use of mental imagery, including hypnotherapy, self-hypnosis and visualization.

Hypnotherapy

Some people still have a cartoon-type image of the hypnotist as a Svengali-like figure with dotted lines coming out of his eyes, intoning: 'You will sleep, you will sleep!' and rendering you unconscious while you obey his will. In fact, a psychologist practising hypnotherapy says, 'There is only one kind of hypnosis — self-hypnosis.'

Under hypnosis you reach that relaxed, dreamy (but not usually unconscious) state in which suggestions can be more readily received by your right brain, bypassing the disbelieving left brain. It has sometimes had remarkable results in healing the physical body, and can be very helpful in the relief of pain. But your mind will only receive those suggestions it is willing to receive.

Hypnotherapy is not a simple process of telling you that you will sleep well, or stop smoking, or eat less. A good hypno-therapist will need to know why you are not sleeping, and will help you to tackle the problems underlying your insomnia, before going on to help you make inner changes to achieve more control over your own behaviour.

Hypnotherapists work in a variety of ways, but will normally start by taking your case history and discussing your current problems. They have their own favourite methods of helping you to relax, perhaps by counting down slowly from ten to one, or by asking you to take yourself in imagination to a peaceful, pleasant place — perhaps a country scene, or the seaside, imagining the sights, colours, scents and sounds.

In this relaxed state, with the logical brain on hold, the therapist can help you review your anxieties and fears in a safe atmosphere. He or she may help you to discover those other, more helpful parts of yourself that have been repressed, and explore ways of making changes in your life. This can be quite an enjoyable game, in which you imagine new scenarios with yourself as both actor and director.

'Hypnotherapy can give you a kind of breathing space,' says hypnotherapist Gloria May, 'so you can stand back from what's going on and view it a bit more objectively. When you go into the alpha state you are more creative and you can often get a handle on things, which is impossible when you're in an overstressed, anxious state.

'Plugging into your unconscious heals the rift between consciousness and unconsciousness, and the more conscious you are the better position you are in to handle more and more. It's not really the stress that makes people insecure, it's the way they see it. Hypnotherapy can be a tremendous help in increasing the level of stress people can handle. It gives you a chance to look at problems in a less emotional way.'

It can be very useful if you suffer from recurrent bad dreams or nightmares. A hypnotherapist can help you to discover what those dreams are trying to tell you, and resolve the tension that keeps them recurring. It is also possible to learn to take an active part in one's dreams and so gain some control over them. Challenging and overcoming a fearful figure or event in a dream can have a big spin-off effect on your self-esteem and ability to control your own destiny.

Hypnotherapy is not an instant answer (there are not too many instant answers, unfortunately) and a number of sessions are usually needed to bring about change. But it can be extremely helpful for insomnia, particularly if the insomniac co-operates by making any other necessary changes to his or her lifestyle and daily habits.

It is important to go to someone who is also an experienced

psychotherapist. Hypnotherapy is a wide-open field with more than 80 training courses, some of them excellent, some of them superficial. Medical hypnotherapists express concern about those without medical training; if someone goes to them for help with headaches or indigestion, believing the symptoms to be stress-induced, it is feared that a serious physical problem may be overlooked. However, a responsible hypnotherapist, medically qualified or not, should ensure that you have had a medical diagnosis before treating you.

Self-hypnosis and visualization

Once their clients are familiar with the experience of reaching a state of hypnosis, most hypnotherapists encourage them to practise self-hypnosis at home; some make tapes for their clients. Many other alternative practitioners also encourage people to use visualization, which is really identical with self-hypnosis, to help their own healing process.

The imagination can have a direct effect on the body, for good or ill. When you imagine or remember a disaster, your pulse can start racing and your breathing can become more shallow, as the body's stress system starts revving up. It doesn't matter that the disaster isn't real: your body and nervous system react as though it is. Similarly, when you imagine yourself healthy and happy, your body starts to feel healthier and stronger.

In a relaxed, day-dreaming state, you can mentally picture the outcome that you want, whether it's better sleep, or confidently taking and passing your driving test. It's important to believe and expect that what you visualize will come about. In so doing, you are using an in-depth way of reprogramming your computer.

Visualization techniques may not be right for everyone: if you are an anxious striver, you may put too much effort into what should be effortless, or make yourself worse by focusing on symptoms rather than health. But even if you don't use specific techniques, you are using the power of thought and imagination throughout the day, both mentally and verbally. All the more reason to exchange depressing thoughts about your life and your sleep for positive ideas about what you really want.

For successful self-hypnosis, the first, essential step is to be able to relax deeply. If you are normally tense, you may need some help in learning to relax sufficiently. (See Part 3, Chapter 2 for more about relaxation.) Some people have successfully taught themselves to visualize from books; there are also some good tapes on the market which can start you off, though it's not a good idea to rely on them for the rest of your life. For most people it's easier initially to be taught by someone else.

A good training course in visualization techniques is the Silva Method, named after its Mexican founder José Silva. The Silva Method is taught over two weekends; starting with learning to relax and enter the alpha-state, it includes techniques for using the whole of your mind, from problem solving, getting to sleep and programming helpful dreams, to healing and the development of ESP. It has helped numbers of people to sleep better, and to give up addictions including alcohol, smoking and tranquillizers.

Thought and energy

Balancing the two hemispheres of the brain can also help to balance the energies of your body. Alternative practitioners and healers in particular, together with a few doctors, are increasingly recognizing that human beings are more than their physical bodies. We also consist of a complete energy system: the energy-field surrounding the body (often referred to as the aura), together with channels of energy flowing through the body and a number of major energy centres (also called chakras) which relate to the endocrine glands.

To feel balanced, harmonious and healthy, the energies within the body need to be flowing harmoniously, without resistance, and the energy field needs to be clear. Negative thoughts, traumas, griefs, stress, can clutter the energy field and clog the channels. In insomnia it seems as if the energies are somehow stuck; changing your thoughts and taking physical action can help to restore the normal, healthy flow.

Although invisible to most people, the energy system can be seen by some psychics and healers, and physically sensed by many healers and natural therapists. Many of those who work directly on the body, like manipulative therapists, massage practitioners and healers, can help to rebalance your energies, and will encourage you to maintain that balance.

The healer Betty Shine stresses the importance of the energy of the mind, which she sees as separate from that around the body. In her book *Mind to Mind* (Corgi, 1989) she describes how, when someone is depressed, the mind energy funnels down like a black cloud, compressing the physical organs and eventually impeding their healthy functioning; conversely, when someone thinks happy, positive thoughts, she can see the mind energy radiating outwards like a halo, lifting depression from the physical system. As you become more self-aware it's possible to sense this for yourself; negative thoughts and unhappiness create a feeling of contraction and constriction, while happiness and optimism make your head and body feel lighter and clearer.

Most healers and health practitioners agree that your thoughts have a direct effect on your body and energy system, which is worth bearing in mind next time you start brooding about something unpleasant. In fact, many go further: thoughts, they say, are forms of energy which, if focused on often enough, will take material form. This helps to explain why people who expect disasters very often get them, and why it's important to exchange negative views of life for positive ones.

Getting help

Some GPs, dentists and psychologists practise hypnotherapy within the Health Service, so it's worth asking your doctor if he or she can refer you to one. Unfortunately they are rather few and far between, and it may be necessary to go privately, which can cost around £30-40 a session, or more. (It's worth it if it changes your life.)

Beware of hypnotists who do not have a psychotherapeutic training. Preferably, find someone through personal recommendation, or through one of the following organizations, enclosing an s.a.e with any written enquiries.

The British Society of Experimental and Clinical Hypnosis,
Secretary, Dr M Heap,
Department of Psychology,
Middlewood Hospital,
Sheffield S6 1TP
Tel. 0742 852222

The British Society of Medical and Dental Hypnosis,
PO Box 6,
42 Links Road,
Ashtead,
Surrey KT21 2HJ
Tel. 03722 73522

The National Council of Psychotherapists
and Hypnotherapy Register,
1 Clovelly Road,
Ealing,
London W5 5HF
Tel. 081 567 0262

The Federation of Hypnotherapists,
10 Alexander Street,
Bayswater,
London W2 5NT
Tel. 071 727 2006

The Institute for Complementary Medicine,
21 Portland Place,
London W1N 3AF
Tel. 071 636 9543
(Has a register of approved hypnotherapists.)

Silva Method courses are given regularly in London and Manchester, and occasionally in other parts of the UK. Details from:
Intermedia,
216 Heaton Moor Road,
Stockport,
Chesire SK4 4DU
Tel. 061 431 0001

Further reading

Dr Vernon Coleman, *Mind Power, How to Use Your Mind to Heal Your Body,* (Century, 1986)
Hellmut W.A. Karle, *Hypnosis and Hypnotherapy, A Patient's Guide,* (Thorsons, 1988)
Matthew Manning's Guide to Self Healing, (Thorsons, 1989)

Guy Lyon Playfair, *Medicine, Mind and Magic*, (Aquarian Press, 1987)

Dr Brian Roet, *All in the Mind? Think yourself better*, (Macdonald Optima, 1987)

Betty Shine, *Mind to Mind*, (Corgi, 1989)

José Silva and Philip Miele, *The Silva Mind Control Method*, (Grafton Books, 1980)

Audio cassettes

A number of cassette tapes are available which can help you relax and reprogramme your thoughts. Some health food shops stock them, and they are usually available at health and Mind, Body and Spirit exhibitions. Since our likes, particularly for voices, are very personal, it is difficult to give blanket recommendations; try to listen before buying.

The healer Matthew Manning has made a complete series of self-help tapes incorporating visualization exercises on a number of subjects, including insomnia and depression. Details from:

The Matthew Manning Centre,
39 Abbeygate Street,
Bury St Edmunds,
Suffolk IP33 1LW
Tel. 0284 69502

CHAPTER 4

The churning mind

Probably the most common complaint among poor sleepers is difficulty in getting off to sleep. It's almost always related to a mind that won't switch itself off. Your thoughts go round and round, you toss and turn, and an hour later you're tired, twitchy, and wide awake.

The churning mind may be caused by anxiety about something specific — an exam, a job interview, a work project, a partner's illness, or the state of your finances. It is possibly caused even more often by resentment or anger, brooding over unpleasant events, sometimes from the recent past, sometimes from way back. You relive the scenes, inventing scenarios in which you find just the right words to put down that person who insulted you yesterday, or even years ago. Or you may be feeling depressed and lonely, wishing your life were different, blaming yourself or others because it isn't, and replaying past regrets, missed opportunities, or lost happiness.

A great deal of night-time churning is connected with unfinished business, something that computer in your head can't stand. It chugs away looking for solutions, and won't shut up. Or it allows you to get to sleep, and then wakes you up with a bad dream to remind you of a problem, or to tell you, 'Hey, we really must do some worrying about this!'

Regularly waking with nightmares or bad dreams can make you anxious about going to bed in the first place; usually these, too, concern unfinished business. Night terrors — suddenly waking from non-dreaming sleep with a sense of fear and doom — are often the result of past traumas. Recurring dreams, too, may stem from traumatic past events — car crashes, a battering spouse, or an assault — which the conscious mind has tried to forget. But the unconscious mind is still trying to cope with it in the only way it knows how. In such cases it is important to seek professional help from a counsellor, psychotherapist or hypnotherapist who can help you to heal your fears, so that they no longer fester and cause you misery.

Some people aren't particularly worried about anything, but just have very active minds. Many of them accept this, often creative people who come up with creative ideas as they lie awake. But if your thoughts are unpleasant, sad or anxious, they are crying out to be dealt with.

Bed is not the place to deal with them.

Who's in the driving seat?

Sometimes we don't know why we feel anxious; some people don't even recognize that they *are* anxious. Hypnotherapist Gloria May points out: 'A lot of chronic insomniacs seem to rush around trying to get themselves tired enough to go to sleep, but it doesn't tie up like that. I think sometimes they are seeking oblivion from problems they're unaware of. The state of going into sleep is when your unconscious chucks things up, and they want to avoid that. But even then, they're often not even aware of worries popping up; they just say "I can't get to sleep".'

Rushing round all day and going to bed with a mind that's exhausted but awake is all too common these days. Modern life doesn't encourage natural rhythms. We start work at the same time all year round, whether it's dark or light; commuter travel is uncomfortable and frustrating. Office atmospheres are often unhealthy as well as fraught; lunch may be a snatched sandwich or hamburger. For many people 'relaxation' takes place in the artificial atmosphere and noise of pubs and discos.

Small wonder that rushers-round can't sleep. The whole physical and nervous system becomes jangled and out of gear. There is no breathing space to look at problems — or just to breathe! Body and mind are poorly nourished. And underlying this frantic rush, an anxious little voice is often sending anxious little messages that we don't want to hear — 'Am I good enough?' — 'Is this all there is to life?' — 'Why aren't I happy?'.

If your life is anything like this, and it has resulted in insomnia, ask yourself what you are truly getting out of it. OK, so modern life is like that. But does that mean *yours* has to be? What or who is driving you to over-work, eat badly, maybe drink too much, or work till all hours so that by bedtime your brain is buzzing?

Much of our busy-busy behaviour is due to conditioning by other people, and our beliefs about how life should be lived may be nothing to do with what we really need. The work ethic says we mustn't waste a moment; social standards say we must have a 'good time' and be successful. We must also be *seen* to be successful by buying and owning more and more goodies for ourselves and our families; to keep the merry-go-round turning we have to work even harder. Yet when you were a child, was it this that you wanted from life? Who programmed your computer?

Our beliefs come from a number of different sources, which is why they often conflict. Some psychotherapists point out that we all have multiple personalities, often referred to as sub-personalities or 'voices'. For example, most people have an inner critic sitting in judgement on their every action; at the same time there's an inner child, made to feel small by the critic's remarks. Many of us have an inner saboteur, doing its best to make us make a mess of things. But there are other parts of us which often don't get a look in — for example, a wise self, a peaceful self, and a creative child who wants to play.

None of these voices are the whole you. But you may be allowing one or a few of them to drive you into more and more activity, because that's what they see as 'leading a full life'. They are kidding you. What they are actually doing is forcing you to drive on one cylinder, heading towards burn-out. To be your whole self, in touch with all your resources, you need to recognize the existence of those other, neglected parts of you. It could be their need to be heard that is keeping you awake.

So, see if you can hear the thoughts and voices underlying your daily rush. Who's driving you on? Are you responding to other people's programming — perhaps a critical father demanding that you prove your worth, or a perfectionist mother setting you impossibly high standards? Do you have to believe those voices from the past? What does the real you need and want from life, and are you getting it?

Depression and sadness

Although it's possible to be both anxious and depressed, usually the last thing a depressed person wants to do is rush around: one of the most common symptoms of depression is lack of energy. Depression comes in many forms and degrees of severity. There are two main types: reactive depression, triggered by unhappy or difficult events, and endogenous depression that can strike some people regularly for no good reason at all. At its worst it becomes clinical depression, which may need medical or psychiatric treatment.

As long as you are not clinically depressed, you can start helping yourself — and the sooner the better, before the habit of depression becomes too ingrained. You will need to make an effort to go against the lethargy that keeps you down. But it really is possible to change your self-denigrating thoughts and feelings about yourself, though you may need some help in doing so.

Depressed people are usually very self-critical. One aspect of depression is feeling that you are such a terrible person you don't deserve to be happy, which can make it difficult to pull yourself out of it. Start listening to your self-talk, and ask yourself whether you would be as hard on anyone else as you are on yourself? You deserve to be happy and fulfilled.

Long-term depression often harks back to childhood. Unloving or over-critical parents have perhaps instilled the message that you are no good, unlovable, or always in the wrong, and the computer obediently repeats these messages. *You don't have to believe them.*

The vast majority of people can learn to feel better about themselves, just as one learns a new skill. But you will have to take the first steps, by deciding to make the change.

Hidden depression

As with anxiety, people don't always know that they are depressed. They may feel constantly tired and lethargic; some people complain they can't concentrate, or that their memory is going. Others may get physical aches and pains, particularly headaches and backaches, or lose their appetite for food or sex. In some, depression disguises itself as anxiety. So if you haven't been able to fathom the cause of your insomnia, could you be concealing unhappiness from yourself?

The 48-year-old wife of an American businessman had suffered from insomnia for several months, despite trying various sleeping pills. When interviewed at a sleep laboratory she said she couldn't think why she wasn't sleeping: for the first time in her life she had everything she had ever wished for and really 'should be happy'.

It took further tests and in-depth interviewing for her to begin to realize what she was really feeling: that for the first time in her life she felt increasingly useless. Her children had left home, some neighbours who had always leaned on her for support had moved, and she felt her life was over, with nothing left for her to do.

Tests in a sleep laboratory showed that she really was sleeping very poorly. She was given an anti-depressant sedative, which helped her to sleep, and with psychotherapy she explored ways of becoming useful again, finally becoming involved in voluntary work for a charity. Nine months later she was off all drugs and her sleep was greatly improved; objective measurements showed that it wasn't perfect, but she was satisfied with the sleep she was getting, as well as with her daily life.*

The unfulfilled mind

Some people, while not depressed or anxious, develop sleep problems because they are simply not doing enough. In his book *Insomnia and other Sleeping Problems* (Sphere Books, 1982) Dr Peter Lambley suggests that rather than being over-stressed, they are not expending enough physical and mental energy during the day to earn themselves deep sleep. This leads to a syndrome he calls malsomnia — light, broken sleep from which you wake up tired. In the malsomniac there is too much light sleep, too many wakenings, and not enough deep and REM sleep.

There can be physical reasons for light, broken sleep, particularly lack of exercise, so a good start to dealing with malsomnia is to ensure that you take regular, physically tiring

*Peter Hauri, Ph.D, *The Sleep Disorders*, (Upjohn, 1977)

exercise. But broken sleep may also be a message that you need to do something about your daytime life. Dr Lambley suggests that sufferers are anxious, nervous people who are afraid of taking risks; over-protective of themselves, they avoid confrontations and challenges. They may be people who try very hard to be 'good', avoiding conflict and therefore only *partly* living. They can also be people who have retired from work that made life meaningful, and instead of enjoying the rest that they looked forward to, feel bored and unfulfilled.

Like the rushers-round, they are not really working towards what they really want, and they are also depriving themselves of the conflicts and challenges that generate REM sleep and dreaming. The inner voices here may be connected with over-protective or over-critical parents. Many people have found it difficult to reach their full potential because a mother or father dealt them the double message: 'It's really important to be a success — but of course, you are not good enough!' Which is enough to immobilize some people for a long time.

Facing up to the problem

Night-time is no time to deal with anxieties, regrets and general unpleasantness. But it may be the only time you've left for them to be heard, because they are uncomfortable. Busy with other things during the day, you brush your worries under the carpet and promise yourself you'll deal with them later. Only you don't. Meanwhile, under the carpet they grow into monsters which creep up on you when you're at your most vulnerable.

It's really vital to deal with that unfinished business during the day. It's not going to go away until you do. Once you start taking some sort of action, even if it's only the decision to take action, the energy that has been stuck, going round in circles, or keeping you depressed, will begin to flow.

Talking to someone else is a good start, whether it's a professional counsellor, your partner or an understanding friend. Airing your troubles begins to get them out of your head, and once they're out they can look far less frightening than when they loom up in the dark hours.

If you're anxious, talking with someone else may help you to realize that anxiety is actually quite normal; other people get anxious, too, and ride it out. Without uncertainties life would be pretty boring. Half the enjoyment of films and books is not knowing how they will end. Anxiety in fact is very akin to excitement. It can spur you to action. It's only when it becomes crippling that anxiety itself is something to worry about.

For depression, too, finding a good listener can help you to get those debilitating feelings out of your system. Don't be ashamed to ask for professional help in the form of counselling or psychotherapy; I'll talk more about this in the next chapter.

For the unfulfilled, talking with someone else can help you to uncover what's holding you back, and help you to move forward.

Meanwhile, if you've no one to talk to, start getting things out of your system by writing them down, or even drawing pictures of them. Some people find it helps to have a teddy bear or a doll to talk to — it may sound childish but it often works. Or keep a 'worry-jar': every time a worry pops into your head, write it on a slip of paper and put it in the jar. (If you wait till it's full to clear it out, you may be surprised at some of the worries in there that no longer seem important at all.)

Change your self-talk

Really listen to your thoughts, and see if you can't change them. Is your anxiety based on reality? Supposing you don't pass that exam, or driving test, or get through that interview, is it really a matter of life or death? What's the worst that can happen? Can you remember a previous time when you were anxious and everything turned out fine?

Similarly, if you are depressed, you are probably regularly feeding yourself negative statements. Remind yourself that they are the result of faulty computer programming. What parents or teachers said about you in the past has nothing to do with the real you, now. Start to talk kindly to yourself, as you would have liked to be talked to when you were a child. Eventually that inner child will begin to feel happier.

Above all, resolve not to focus on your depression. It may hang around you like a cloud, which makes it difficult to ignore, but you don't have to get sucked into it. Try to regard it as you would regard bad weather; it's making the world look grey for the moment, but it will pass. Meanwhile, it doesn't have to stop you living life to the full.

If your inner voices tell you you're too depressed to go out and see people, or take a walk on a pleasant day, you don't have to obey them. If you start acting contrary to their commands, you'll be showing them who's boss. And you will also be unlocking that locked-up energy so that it can start flowing healthily again.

Take some action

Whether you're anxious, depressed or unfulfilled, it's important to start moving. The longer you put off doing something about an unsatisfactory situation, the worse it gets — and the more your mind will churn when you get to bed. Energy that you could be using during the day revolves in circles, keeping you unhappy and uncomfortable, instead of being used creatively. When you start to move forward, that energy will support you. There's more about the kinds of changes you can make in Part 3; meanwhile, if you have a particular problem or anxiety that you've been putting off facing, start now!

Dealing with specific problems

If you're being kept awake by specific problems, learn to deal with them during the day, so that you don't take unfinished business to bed with you.

Find some time during the day or early evening to write a list of the worries or anxieties that are keeping you awake. A friend of mine who did this realized she had one 'super-anxiety', around which revolved a set of sub-anxieties. Once she'd taken steps to deal with the super-anxiety, many of the sub-anxieties were automatically cleared up, and the rest became much less important.

Having identified the super-anxiety, write down what you can do about it. If you're worried about a job interview, what steps can you take to prepare yourself for it? If getting a job interview is difficult, what can you do about it? Are there any alternatives to the kind of action you've been taking so far?

Once you've decided on your course of action, close your eyes for a few minutes and see yourself taking it. If you are anxious about a forthcoming event, or finally doing that thing you've been nervous about, picture yourself dealing with it calmly and efficiently; don't imagine all the difficulties in the way, but see the successful end-product. Set the scene very clearly: see yourself with your problem solved or having achieved the thing you fear doing. Imagine telling someone about it, and hearing their congratulations. Don't worry if you can't visualize clearly; imagine how you'll feel — relieved, pleased with yourself, no longer anxious. In this way you are priming your brain with the fact that solutions are possible; anxiety or hesitation are not the only options.

Then close your notebook, and put it in a drawer for the night, knowing *you have done everything you can*. Physically putting your list away tells the anxious or worried part of your mind that that's it for today, thank you! You are also making space for the more creative part of your mind to come up with solutions, possibly during sleep.

Then, having identified what action to take, *do it!* It's amazing how anxiety and fear disappear and depression lifts when you actually get going on a project. The mind can't focus on two things at once. Actors who suffer from stagefright lose it when they walk on the stage and begin concentrating on their roles. If you are really involved in and concentrated on an activity, there isn't room for negative feelings.

Supposing, for some reason, there is no direct action you can take to deal with the problem itself? *What you can do right now* is to take physical action to deal with your state of anxiety, depression or lethargy.

Looking after your body

Anxiety, depression, and obsessive thinking all have a strong physical component, since they trigger the production of stress hormones which create further anxiety, depression and obsessive thinking. Breaking the cycle by looking after your body will have a positive feedback on your emotions.

Stress hormones are actually produced to gear us up for action. If you start taking regular exercise you will get rid of them healthily. You have to make a commitment, says my 'super-anxiety' friend; part of her strategy was to go swimming every day. She had to force herself to go to the pool for the first few days, but it was worth it; feeling physically relaxed and well helped her to get back in control.

I'll be going more fully into looking after the body in Parts 3 and 4, but meanwhile, remember that:

— Caffeine can keep the mind churning, and in some people causes depression and anxiety.

— Smoking also over-stimulates the nervous system.

— Alcohol may lift your mood short-term; long-term it depletes the adrenal glands and can make you more anxious or depressed.

— Lack of exercise allows a build-up of stress hormones that result in anxiety and depression.

— Learning to relax physically helps you to relax mentally. It's quite hard to be relaxed and feel anxious or unhappy at the same time. (See Part 3.)

— Check whether environmental stress is making you feel worse; read the section on Geopathic Stress in Chapter 8.

Natural therapies

Some forms of depression are physically based — post-flu and post-natal depression, for instance. Anxiety and depression in themselves deplete your energies, and become exaggerated when your general health is below par.

Most forms of natural medicine help to lift the emotions as well as healing the body. Homoeopathy, herbalism, and acupuncture can help to restore your emotional balance; so can bodywork, perhaps combined with counselling, from a massage practitioner or aromatherapist. Spiritual healing works on all levels, calming and uplifting body and mind.

It's worth trying osteopathy, incidentally, for post-natal depression; the sacrum (the shield-like bone at the bottom of the spine) can be displaced by pregnancy and giving birth, and some osteopaths believe that this can have a profound effect on the balance of your emotions.

As temporary props, herbal tranquillizers are effective and have no harmful side effects. Herbal infusions can be even more helpful, supplying trace elements and minerals that strengthen the nervous system.

Bach Flower Remedies can bring about a totally natural change in your thoughts and feelings. White chestnut, for instance, is good for obsessive thoughts, and mustard for depression. Agrimony, for people who put on a cheerful front concealing inner torment, has helped a number of people recover their sleep.

CHAPTER 5

Someone to talk to

Whether you suffer from anxiety, depression or some other form of unhappiness, there's an awful lot you can do to help yourself, but that doesn't mean that you have to do it *all* yourself. Bottling up your feelings inside keeps them on the churn. Just talking with someone who's sympathetic but objective can release some of that bottled-up energy.

Friends and partners can be a great support, but sometimes people who know you well try to cheer you up or change the subject, when what you really want is a listening, receptive ear. Friends and relations can also feel uncomfortable when they hear you aren't happy, and may tell you that of course you don't *really* feel that way, and all you need to do is to pull yourself together. This is not helpful. Sometimes, of course, they are the cause of your problems, and you find it hard to tell them what's on your mind.

Don't be embarrassed about seeking help from a counsellor or psychotherapist, or feel there's something shameful about needing such help. There really isn't. After all, nobody feels embarrassed at consulting an expert about their finances or buying a new car. Why should you worry about seeing an expert on that priceless item, your emotional health? Getting help in order to help yourself is a much healthier option than staying miserable.

Many personal problems can be helped by short-term counselling. There are cases when psychotherapy can be helpful, when the person hasn't got over traumatic childhood events, for instance. Some people feel that seeing a psychotherapist may be opening a whole can of worms, and they'd rather not, thank you. But if you are sitting on a can of worms, really it's better out than in! Otherwise they simply go on niggling at you.

Psychotherapy doesn't necessarily mean years of delving into the painful past. It's true that how we deal with life and relate to other people is affected by our past. But the purpose of psychotherapy is to change our reactions in the present. (Some psychotherapists and natural practitioners use a technique called Voice Dialogue, which enables all those inner voices to be heard, which in itself can alter your perceptions of yourself, and is also fun.)

Nor will you be putting yourself in the hands of someone who'll take over your life and tell you what to do. A good counsellor or therapist will accept you as you are, for who you are, and listen to you in a way that people who are involved with you may not be able to. Being really heard will help you to listen to yourself and understand yourself in a new way. As you begin to unburden your mind of problems, you can begin to find your own solutions.

That said, the field of psychotherapists and counsellors contains both good therapists and bad. I have heard complaints that some psychotherapists do keep their clients in a subservient role, putting them in the wrong or making them feel inadequate. If you start therapy with anyone like this, just leave. These people are also quite skilled at making you feel guilty when you announce you are leaving; don't let them. It's your life, and a therapist's job is to make you feel more whole, not smaller.

How do you set about finding this kind of help? Here are some of the sources you could try:

Your doctor:

Some GPs are very aware of the value of counselling, and are good at it themselves when they have the time. Some are in touch with local counselling services to whom they can refer you. They can also refer you to psychiatrists or clinical psychologists within the National Health Service.

Other doctors, alas, are less clued up; you can still ask them to get you an appointment with your local hospital psychiatric or psychological medicine department.

Psychiatrists:

They have a medical training and can prescribe drugs if they feel it necessary, which isn't always the case. To a normally anxious person, for example, some may recommend relaxation training, or meditation. Some may refer you on to a psychologist; some have themselves taken additional trainings in subjects like hypnotherapy or psychotherapy.

Clinical psychologists:

They work within the NHS and are not doctors, but are trained in helping with emotional problems. They may have a number of techniques to offer, from practical advice to psychotherapy. A popular form of therapy these days is cognitive therapy, aimed at helping people to change a negative self-image by identifying and changing the ways you talk to yourself (along the lines suggested in the previous chapters).

Unfortunately, there are not too many clinical psychologists around; there are only some 1800-2000 in the country. Whether you can get a speedy appointment depends on their availability in your part of the country; in some areas there is a one-year waiting list. But it's worth trying.

Your local church:

Churches and other religious organizations can put you in touch with trained counsellors.

A large number of therapists operate privately, with a wide range of fees. Few of them are cheap, but some counselling services have a sliding scale. With others, it is sometimes possible to see a therapist in his or her final year of training who will charge lower fees than fully qualified therapists.

The best way to choose one is through personal recommendation from a friend, doctor or alternative practitioner. If you have to find one on your own, there are further possible sources of information, including:

Your local Citizen's Advice Bureau

Your local Social Services department

The British Association for Counselling, 37a Sheep Street, Rugby, CV21 3BX, tel. 0788 78328, which has a large register of counsellors and psychotherapists throughout the country. Send an s.a.e. for a list of therapists in your area, together with their qualifications.

The Yellow Pages. A number of psychotherapists and counsellors advertise in the Yellow Pages of the telephone directory. You can always ring up and ask what sort of services they provide. Although this looks a little like taking pot luck, people who advertise in this way are at least successfully in business! You have a right to ask to meet them and chat with them to see how you get on before committing yourself; most therapists also prefer to do this. After all, it's important that you go to someone you like and trust. You also have the right to ask them about their training and qualifications. If they object to your asking, this may well be a sign that they're not for you.

Holistic Health Clinics often have counsellors on their staff.

Health Food Shops sometimes advertise counselling/therapy services; or the manager may be able to give you a personal recommendation.

Natural Health Practitioners. These days more and more complementary or alternative practitioners are recognizing the value of counselling. Some are good intuitive counsellors, and some take further training in counselling on top of their other qualifications.

Other organizations offering help or sources of help include:

The Cruse Club,
Cruse House,
126 Sheen Road,
Richmond,
Surrey TW9 1UR
Tel. 081 940 4818
(The national organization for the widowed and their children.)

Depressives Anonymous,
36 Chestnut Avenue,
Beverley,
Humberside HU17 9QU
Tel. 0482 860619
(A support organization for depressives.)

MIND (National Association for Mental Health),
22 Harley Street,
London W1N 2ED
Tel. 071 637 0741
(It publishes a wide range of literature on all aspects of mental health.)

Relate (formerly the National Marriage Guidance Council),
Herbert Gray College,
Little Church Street,
Rugby,
Warwickshire
Tel. 0788 73241

The Samaritans provide listening ears all over the country; you don't have to be suicidal to phone them. Your local branch will be listed in your telephone directory.

Helpful reading

David Burns, *Feeling Good*, (Signet Press, 1983). (A guide to cognitive therapy)

Anne Dickson, *A Woman in Your Own Right*, (Quartet Press, 1982). (A guide to self-assertion)

Tony Lake, *Living With Grief*, (Sheldon Press, 1984). (A self-help guide to dealing with bereavement and loss)

Andrew Stanway, *Defeating Depression*, (Arrow Books, 1987). (A guide to depression, its medical treatment, and self-help)

Dr Clive Wood, *Living in Overdrive*, (Fontana Paperbacks, 1984). (A guide to reducing stress)

CHAPTER 6

Your sleep and other people

As I mentioned earlier, some sleep experts believe that anger and resentment are more common causes of night-time churning than anxiety or depression. If that's the case with you, it's important to drop them, for the sake of your sleep. It is possible!

If you're angry about a current situation, either accept it or do something about it; otherwise all that negative energy (and there's a lot of energy in anger) will go on keeping you awake.

Many people fear confrontations, but it is possible to say what you feel about a situation without having a violent explosion. Telling the person or people concerned calmly how you feel about their behaviour, without blaming or accusing them, can often open up better communications.

If you can't confront the person, or if the anger-making situation is in the past, whether it's last week or several years ago, tell yourself that whatever anybody else has said or done, however unfair, cruel, snide, or dishonest, it's over now. While you are brooding, going over the scene or scenes, rehearsing the remarks you could have made, or intend to make in the future, the other person may well have forgotten the whole thing. The only person who's making you angry now is you, every time you mentally relive those scenes.

In addition, if you accept the suggestion that thought is energy, consider this: what we think comes back to us. It is generally accepted in healing and spiritual groups that when we send thoughts of healing and kindness to other people, not only will those people benefit but so will we. Thoughts of resentment and vengeance may not affect other people at all, unless it's to make them even more unpleasant; but they most certainly will boomerang back at us.

A young woman was persuaded by a friend to take the Silva Method course, though she wasn't too keen. She had been going through a bad time. She hadn't been able to sleep without pills since a car accident, and she was also full of vengeance towards her ex-husband. When her friend told her her vengeful thoughts would attract negativity to herself, she dismissed the idea as rubbish. However, during the course, she began to understand the sense of it. After regularly practising the techniques, including forgiving her husband, her life has become happier, she sleeps well without pills, and is amazed at the happy relationship she has with her ex-husband; she has also developed powers of healing.

There are other considerations in storing anger. You are not only keeping yourself awake. Firstly, you are setting yourself up for physical problems: high blood pressure, heart problems and arthritis are among the side-effects of long-harboured anger. Secondly, when you let someone else's behaviour rule your thoughts, emotions and sleep, you are making the person responsible for your peace of mind, handing over to them your personal autonomy.

So, anger and resentment and all those feelings of 'it's not fair' are best dropped. I know that's easier said than done. But once you really see that they're doing you no good, you can at least decide to let them go. This decision is the first step towards freedom; it will set your thoughts moving in a different direction.

Resentment is often a deeply ingrained habit, but it's one we may have been taught by others. Small children are naturally forgiving; I suspect that some of us learn to be resentful from our elders. It's an unhealthy habit, and once you've given it up you will feel better all round.

Do try to get it physically out of your system, during the day. Anger creates the tense muscles that give you headaches and shoulder pain, as well as stimulating the release of stress hormones, all of which can contribute to your insomnia.

One way is the famous pillow-bashing technique, which really does work. Find a time and a place where you can be alone, and make a pillow the focus of your anger. Don't think of it as the person you are angry with: you are not trying to hurt anyone else but to heal yourself. Start thumping. Yell at the same time. Really let go, and keep shouting and thumping until you are exhausted, drained of your angry feelings, and with your shoulders and arms released of all that tension.

If punching pillows is not your scene, there are other options, like driving to a lonely spot and shouting at the top of your voice. Or write a letter to the person who's bugging you and then tear it up and burn it. Get all the exercise you can, particularly exercise which uses your arm muscles.

The next stage is to forgive the person or people in question. That can be a hard one, but the important thing is your willingness to forgive. Forgiveness doesn't mean that you condone bad behaviour, or that you have to let anyone continue to treat you badly; it means that you are wiping your own slate clean and getting the past out of your system.

Visualization techniques can be helpful here. In a relaxed state you can visualize the other person, possibly attached to you by cords that your thoughts and feelings have created. See yourself cutting through those cords and burning them, freeing you both. Or imagine a conversation in which you tell the person that you're releasing them from your thoughts. It may help to imagine them apologizing to you!

Another approach is to imagine your mind as a beautiful room, in which you have the right to entertain the guests of your choice. At the moment it's full of these cross, grumbling people, reminding you you've been hard done by. Tell them you don't enjoy their company, and show them the door. If they're reluctant to leave, sweep them out with a broom! Your room is now empty and clean, and there is space in it for more welcome visitors, including peace of mind, serenity and better sleep. Show them in and make them at home.

You may have to repeat these exercises several times before your brain really accepts the message. But although it may take a little time, so long as you have a genuine commitment to forgiving and letting go, you will find yourself becoming truly free of these past resentments.

A lot of depressed people suffer from guilt and anger towards themselves, quite often for no good reason. If you belong to this group, do be kind to yourself. Forgive yourself as you would forgive anyone else. Use visualization to let go of those feelings and start afresh, reminding yourself of all the good things about you.

Sometimes anger and resentment are so deeply rooted that people need help in sorting them out — if their parents neglected or ill-treated them in childhood, for instance. In that case, do get some professional counselling. Of course, it's usually easier to forgive someone who's not around than the person playing records upstairs all night — or snoring beside you in bed.

Partnership problems

Most marriages and partnerships go through bad patches; feeling resentful towards your partner can be a major source of sleeplessness. Do try to resolve your problems, or at least start to, during the day or early evening: don't leave it until bedtime to have rows. And don't lie in bed brooding over your partner's faults and telling yourself that if only he or she were different you would be quite happy.

You cannot change other people; what you can do is to tell them how you feel — they may have no idea. And give them the opportunity to tell you how they feel. People often make totally false assumptions about what's going on in someone else's head, even their nearest and dearest. Talking openly and honestly, and listening to the other person's point of view as well as expressing your own, can clear the air remarkably at times.

Women often have difficulty in acknowledging that they are angry at all; we are still brought up with the idea that anger isn't very nice. Some women repress their own wants and needs in order to be perfect wives and mothers; they don't realize that underneath they are quite angry at constantly giving out to others. This kind of situation can trigger insomnia. If you are constantly giving out to others, make sure that you get your own needs met as well.

It has been found helpful for couples to have a regular weekly date and time for expressing their grievances in turn, and listening to each other without interruption while they are expressed. End the session by telling your partner what you appreciate about them; couples often neglect this. You hear people say, 'I don't have to tell my wife/husband I love her/him, she/he knows without me telling her/him.' I think that's an awful pity. It doesn't matter whether we know or not, it's always heart-warming to be told.

When you live with someone else it can be a good idea to have a spare bed ready made up, or a sofa, to which one of you can retire when you both need space. (Don't retire to it forever, though, if you want to keep the relationship going.)

In some of the books and articles I've read about insomnia, the writers remark gaily that sex is the one activity it's good to indulge in before bedtime, the assumption being that you then drop off, happy and relaxed.

What if you don't? An unsatisfactory sexual relationship can leave at least one partner feeling worse off than with no sex at all. As with all the other problems causing insomnia, it's important to do something about it. The longer difficulties build up the more insoluble they can seem.

If you have a good relationship and goodwill on both sides, and if your partner agrees, ask your doctor to put you in touch with a sex therapist (unfortunately they're not easily available on the NHS), or get in touch with a marriage guidance counsellor. If there's no real goodwill, of course, you need to ask yourself why you are staying in this marriage. Again, it can be helpful to see a marriage guidance or some other kind of counsellor, to help you to clarify the confused feelings that are keeping you awake.

Even in a good relationship, there's usually room for improvement. Many men don't realize that physical contact doesn't have to lead to sex, and studiously ignore their partners if they don't feel like performing. Meanwhile, the woman may be longing for a friendly cuddle. Learning to touch each other in non-sexual ways, perhaps by taking a massage course together, can do a lot for your relationship and your sleep.

Noisy neighbours

Meanwhile, what about those neighbours thumping about upstairs or next door? They can be infuriating, and getting infuriated is going to keep you awake just as much as the noise. If it's really horrendous, with regular all-night parties, for instance, you can complain to the police, who may or may not be helpful, your local authority (some of whom are helpful about asking noisy neighbours to keep it down), or your Environmental Health Officer.

Very often the trouble lies as much with bad soundproofing,

particularly in flats, as with the noisy neighbours. The construction of some buildings actually magnifies noise, and the people making it may have no idea that they are disturbing you.

If you can't do anything about improving your soundproofing and the noise is consistent, tell the neighbours about it, *unaggressively.* If you don't already know them, forming friendly relations with the person who is thumping above your head or next door makes the disturbance much less threatening and therefore more bearable.

Try to keep a sense of humour and think of other possible solutions. A friend of mine, woken every night by a pair of high heels clomping about on an uncarpeted floor, presented their owner with a pair of moccasins, which she wore at night from then on, to the benefit of my friend's sleep.

Ear-plugs can be quite helpful; so can creating your own kind of background noise. Listening to soothing music through headphones usually blocks out other sounds. I often record radio plays, so that if I am kept awake at least I can listen to something I have chosen to hear.

Your attitude can make a lot of difference to how badly you are disturbed. Our sensitivity to noise varies; some people can sleep through a hurricane, but wake when their baby cries. Babies themselves seem to be able to sleep through anything. And my cat will sleep contentedly through other people's parties; she isn't telling herself that she's being disturbed by nasty, inconsiderate people.

The next time noise starts up just as you are going to sleep, give yourself a choice: you can get angry and tense, or you can treat it as a challenge. Try simply living through the noise without attaching to it any emotional thoughts about other people's selfishness. Relax your body, breathe deeply and regularly; know that you are getting the physical rest you need, and congratulate yourself on not getting worked up.

CHAPTER 7

Babies and children

The arrival of a new baby is bound to cause a disruption of sleep, though hopefully a welcome one. Parents who accept that their sleep will be broken while the baby needs night-time feeds suffer less from fatigue than those who feel resentful about it; feeling irritable about losing sleep will lose you more sleep, and will convey itself to the baby. But there is no doubt that this is a tiring period, particularly for mothers. If possible, take time during the day to catnap or simply relax.

Children can suffer from disturbed sleep too, which disturbs parents' sleep in turn. There's nothing like a screaming baby or a bedtime battle with an older child, to create irritability and taut nerves, which will affect you during the day as well as at night.

During the 1980s a number of sleep disorders clinics were started to help the parents of small children suffering from sleep disturbances. Children's needs vary as much as adults, and parents are not always certain whether they are doing the right thing. Nowadays we are beginning to accept that being a parent is an art that not everyone possesses by instinct, and parents feel less defensive than they used to about asking for expert advice.

Sleep clinic advice is always geared to the individual. Very often parents believe that their baby or child has a sleep problem because they have expectations of what the norm should be. But within the 'norm' there are many variations. Some small babies naturally sleep less than the average, without necessarily having a problem. Nor is there anything necessarily wrong if your baby is not acting as the books tell you to expect at its age, or if your neighbour's baby sleeps right through the night when yours doesn't. You may have to work out a routine based on your own needs and the child's.

The subject of sleep in children demands more space than I can give it here. For practical advice on establishing a good sleeping and waking routine and dealing with specific problems, I suggest you read *My Child Won't Sleep*, by two child specialists; clinical psychologist Jo Douglas, and psychiatrist Dr Naomi Richman.

I am sorry, however, that although generally not in favour of giving drugs to children the authors suggest that diazepam, for example, might occasionally be prescribed for children with night terrors or in emergencies. If you have to give a child a sedative, there are equally effective, non-chemical, herbal or homoeopathic remedies. Children also respond very well indeed to Bach Flower Remedies.

Establishing a good routine

Parents can be of tremendous help in laying down a good sleep pattern for their child in the future. A regular, consistent routine helps the child to understand that it is bedtime (small children aren't aware of time), and should be established as early as possible.

Sometimes mothers and babies get off to a bad start when the baby falls asleep on the breast after feeding and learns to associate falling asleep with mother being there. As the child gets old enough to demand your presence, you can teach him or her firmly but lovingly to sleep alone. A firm tone of voice will help to get the message home. Make sure the child has comforting toys, and reassure it that you are around by looking in every now and again, but don't let the habit of only sleeping with you there continue. Above all, be consistent, so that the child learns what to expect.

Bedtime should be a pleasant and enjoyable experience for both parent and child, accompanied by story-telling and plenty of cuddles. It's a good idea for both parents to be involved, perhaps taking it in turns to put the child to bed, so that it doesn't become dependent on the presence of just one of you. From the age of two, it's possible to discuss with your child any problems in settling down or getting up in the night: you can set targets and have a reward system for an uninterrupted night. Try not to have a row with your child just before bedtime. And never send the child to bed as a punishment.

If your child consistently has trouble with getting to sleep, staying asleep or other disturbances, it's useful to keep a sleep diary, as is suggested at sleep disorders clinics and described in *My Child Won't Sleep*. In this you keep a note of what's going on during the day, as well as the hours that the child sleeps, or fails to. You can then observe whether there is a pattern. Do regular nightmares occur, for instance, when father works late? Or is there some other disruption to the daily routine which might be causing anxiety to the child — or yourself? Children very easily pick up when a parent is anxious or worried, and can develop all sorts of ideas about what might be going on, including believing that family problems are somehow all their fault.

Some common sleeping problems

The screaming baby

A screaming baby can be exhausting for both parents and child. There may be a number of reasons for it, and it is a good idea to check that there is nothing physically wrong.

In the first few months a very common cause is colic. It is said that nothing can be done about this, and parents find themselves walking up and down during the night holding the baby until it quietens. However, colic can be helped by some natural medicines, as can other causes of screaming. (See the section of natural therapies towards the end of this chapter.) Gently stroking a small baby's feet is also very soothing and calming.

The colicky stage is a risk area for establishing a pattern of 'baby cries — mother comes running'. While it needs comforting at this time, once the colic is over is the time to get it into the habit of sleeping without expecting parents to be in constant attendance.

The overtired child

Some small children need more sleep than their parents realize; if your child is fractious, particularly at bedtime, it could be overtired. Remember, toddlers don't know what the time is, and it's up to you to tell them firmly that it's bedtime.

Try putting the child to bed earlier; you will soon find out if they benefit from more sleep. But if you do experiment with different bedtimes, give the experiments time to work, so that the child has a chance to adapt to the new routine. A major cause of disturbed sleep patterns in children is inconsistency on the parents' part.

The child who needs less sleep

As children get older, they are sometimes packed off to bed long before they're ready for sleep, because the parents want the evening to themselves. It is confusing for them and their body clocks to be told it is time to sleep when they don't feel sleepy, and they may raise strong objections.

It's best to be honest with them about your own needs. Rather than engaging in a battle, let them play or read in bed until they are ready for sleep. (As a child sent to bed before I was sleepy, I used to read for hours under the bedclothes, to the detriment of my eyesight.) If you trust your child, he or she will go to sleep when they need to. They are less likely to if it becomes a major issue.

Demanding attention in the night

Some children have the parent-debilitating habit of waking in the night and demanding attention. This could be because bad habits have been set up in babyhood when an over-anxious mother has looked in at the slightest sound. Or it could be because they feel they're not getting enough of her attention during the day. But so long as they are getting all the daytime love they need, they could be testing how far they have you on a string.

Providing there is nothing genuinely wrong with them, the standard advice is to leave them to cry, but many parents feel uncomfortable about this. There is a difference, however, in the sound of a child crying simply to get attention, and the cry of a child who is genuinely afraid or unhappy. It may be necessary to show the child you are there, but also let it know what your limits are, kindly but firmly. Leave the child with plenty of toys to play with if it does waken in the night. Again, you could create

a system of rewards, or perhaps a star-chart, for undisturbed
nights.

Sleepwalking

Sleepwalking is quite common in children and adolescents, and
normally tails off in the late teens. It usually occurs in the deep
stages of sleep and the child is not aware of it. It may be a sign
of minor unresolved anxiety, but if it happens regularly there
could be a deeper emotional cause. If occurrences coincide with
particular incidents or some anxiety affecting the child or the
whole family, the child may be in need of reassurance.

Otherwise, don't worry the child by making too much of it. He
or she will normally return to bed spontaneously; don't waken
them. But do make sure there's no danger of the child falling out
of windows or otherwise getting hurt.

Nightmares

Most small children go through a phase of having nightmares,
usually around the ages of three or four, coinciding with a phase
in their development when they are more anxious in general,
and perhaps scared of the dark. If the child remembers the
nightmare next day, he or she may perhaps be frightened of
going to sleep.

Unless they occur very often, nightmares don't necessarily
mean that the child is emotionally disturbed; they can be
triggered by a television programme or the sight of a fierce dog
in the park, for instance. All the same, it's important to respect
the child's fears, and listen to anything they want to tell you
about their dream.

Make the child feel as secure as possible, and let them know
that you are there if needed. They may like to have a nightlight;
you can also appoint a favourite toy as a guardian. Some parents
have helped children to lose their fear of nightmares by getting
them to draw pictures of them and making a game of it — for
example, drawing a dream monster and then putting a red nose
on it. If a child suffers regularly from nightmares, there may be
some deeper cause, and you should talk to your GP about it.

Night terrors

Night terrors occur most often in small children, though adults can experience them too. When they happen the child suddenly sits up in bed, staring into space and screaming in apparent terror. Although these episodes can be very frightening for parents the child usually doesn't remember them. They occur during the deep stages of sleep and are not related to dreams or nightmares. Stay with the child and comfort it until it falls asleep again.

Night terrors may be caused by the child going to bed feeling angry or distressed, and again, if they are frequent, the child may be reacting to some deeper worry or family problem about which it needs reassurance.

Further information

Sleep clinics

Sleep clinics for parents are mainly run by clinical psychologists; some health visitors are also trained in their methods. Many parents find that two or three visits to a sleep clinic, at weekly or fortnightly intervals, are enough to help them sort out problems and uncertainties; serious problems can take a little longer. 'We often get parents saying "If only we'd heard about you sooner!"' says a clinical psychologist in charge of a clinic. 'Often problems get severe which could have been dealt with more easily if they'd been tackled earlier.'

For details of sleep disorders clinics for parents, ask your GP or health visitor.

The Cry-sis Support Group

This group runs a network of self-help telephone contacts and provides an information pack for parents whose babies and children cry incessantly or have sleeping problems. There is a small annual membership fee. Details from:
BM Crysis,
London WC1N 3XX
Tel. 071 404 5011

The Parent Network

Your child's sleeping patterns, like your own, can be a reflection of what's going on during the day. The Parent Network runs groups for parents who recognize that parenting skills aren't all instinctive, and who want to learn to relate better with their children; details from them at 44-46 Caversham Road, London NW5 2DS, tel. 071 485 8535. Its director Ivan Sokolov and journalist Deborah Hutton have written a helpful book on the subject, *The Parents Book*, (Thorsons, 1988).

Natural therapies for children

As I've already mentioned, natural remedies can often soothe an upset child. To help a child get off to sleep herbal drinks and baths can be very soothing; so can massaging a baby's or child's feet. Babies and children also respond very well to Bach Flower Remedies; a few drops of Rescue Remedy or Rock Rose are ideal for a child awoken by a nightmare.

It's possible that allergies are over-diagnosed by some over-enthusiastic natural practitioners. You should be cautious of following very extreme diets in young children. But allergies do occur, very often to cow's milk, as well as to other allergens like food additives. Symptoms include constant upset stomachs, eczema, asthma, hyperactivity, and unexplained misery. If you suspect an allergy, seek advice from a well-qualified homoeopath, naturopath or medical herbalist. Allergic reactions can also sometimes respond to treatments other than diet, such as cranial osteopathy or acupuncture. If you are breast-feeding, check your own diet: a breast-feeding mother who drinks a great deal of tea or coffee will be passing the caffeine on to her baby.

Sometimes babies or toddlers are fractious because they are in physical discomfort; the cause is not always evident to GPs, but it may be something that can be put right relatively easily by an alternative practitioner, a homoeopath or cranial osteopath for instance.

If a baby is ailing or miserable for no evident reason, do ensure that the cot is not in a geopathically stressed area (see the next chapter).

Manipulative techniques

Some osteopaths and chiropractors have a particular interest in treating children and quite small babies; manipulative treatments have cured cases of bed-wetting (when caused by a spinal maladjustment) and even allergies and colic.

Sometimes the actual birth causes a slight maladjustment in the bones of the skull, creating physical discomfort which leads to apparently inexplicable crying. This can be put right very easily by cranial osteopathy. You may even be able to correct it yourself. The test is to take the baby's feet and bring them up over its head: most babies enjoy this and often laugh. If your baby doesn't find it amusing, there could be something awry. The surprisingly simple remedy is to hold the infant upside down by its feet, and swing it, very gently, for a minute or two; again, most babies enjoy this. Since the bones of a baby's skull are quite mobile, the weight of its head is often enough to settle them into their normal position. If this doesn't work, however, do seek professional advice.

Homoeopathy

Children seem naturally to want to be in balance, says a homoeopath. Their systems are quite sensitive and any trauma — mental, physical, emotional or dietary — can knock them slightly out of kilter. Very often a homoeopath can restore the balance by administering a single remedy.

Vaccination can produce after-effects in children more often than is generally realized. These can take the form of eczema, rashes, or chronic catarrhal coughs. Homoeopathy can clear these up, as well as many childhood infections which, if treated with antibiotics, tend to recur time and again. Since homoeopathy affects the mental and emotional levels, it can also help with night-time fears, nightmares and so on.

Other natural treatments particularly suited to children include medical herbalism, the Metamorphic Technique and spiritual healing.

CHAPTER 8

A healthy environment

As has already been mentioned, your bedroom should be associated with sleep, and not with other activities. It should also be warm and welcoming, with a peaceful and healthy atmosphere; some bedrooms, as will be seen the next section, can actually damage your health.

Colours
Colours have an influence not only on our visual sense but on our nervous system; they radiate at different wavelengths, some of which are stimulating, and some calming. Calming colours for bedrooms are soft blues and greens, pastel pinks and peaches; neutral colours like beige and cream are also appropriate. Avoid vivid colours, particularly in a child's bedroom, where they might seem cheerful but can be over-stimulating.

The bed
Your bed should obviously be comfortable, ideally with a firm but not over-hard mattress. People's tastes in mattresses vary, and if you're happy with a squashy one, that's fine. But soft mattresses are not good for your back in the long run.

It's best to sleep with a single pillow, which keeps your neck at a natural angle. A stiff neck is often greatly improved when two or three pillows are replaced with a single one. (It's been suggested, incidentally, that if you sleep badly in strange houses, taking a familiar pillow with you will provide the link with home that will allow sleep to come.) Some people find hop- or herb-filled pillows help them to sleep; you can get them at herbalists like Culpeper's. Sniff before buying to make sure you like the smell.

Fresh, clean air

Fresh air is important, provided it doesn't make the room too cold. If you don't like sleeping with an open window, consider getting an ioniser. Ionisers replace in the atmosphere negative ions, electrically charged molecules which are found in abundance in mountain air and around waterfalls, and which keep the air healthy and clean. (A selection is available from The Ioniser Centre, 65 Endell Street, London WC2, tel. 071 379 7323.)

Crystals

Crystals are getting very popular these days as aids to healing, meditation, and clearing the atmosphere. Rose quartz and amethyst are both suitable stones for sleep; keep one by your bedside. When you buy a crystal, it should be thoroughly cleansed before you use it, since crystals absorb energies from the atmosphere around them. Soak it for several hours in a bowl of salt water, rinse it under the cold tap, don't wipe it with a cloth but place it to dry on a sunny window sill.

Is your bedroom healthy?

Over the last few years complaints of headaches, skin rashes, nausea, lethargy, depression, stress and fatigue have been related to 'sick building syndrome'. The health of workers in modern buildings has been affected by factors like artificial lighting, static electricity from synthetic furniture and fabrics, low frequency electromagnetic radiation from electronic machinery, and airborne particles. Air-conditioning and non-openable windows further deplete the atmosphere of negative ions.

We don't hear too much about 'sick bedrooms', but some of these factors can also affect your home, particularly if you are sensitive. Though it's unlikely that your bedroom will be full of computers, an increasing number of synthetic fabrics are used in furnishings, bedlinen and nightwear, while harmful gas can be given off by insulation materials, lacquers, glues and vinyls. There is also increasing evidence that radiation from electric pylons can affect the health of people living near them.

So, use natural fabrics in your bedroom furnishings, linen and nightwear; and don't have a TV set in there. Although single items of electrical and electronic equipment are said to give off safe levels of radiation, we are increasingly exposed to radiation of all kinds, and the accumulation from various sources can ultimately get to us. It's also best not to use an electric blanket; if you do, switch it off and unplug it before going to bed.

There is another cause of 'sick bedrooms' which has only recently started to receive publicity here, though in the United States and Germany scientists and doctors are very aware of it. And that is geopathic stress.

Geopathic stress

I used to think that ley lines, the lines of electromagnetic energy running through the earth, were of strictly academic or hippy interest — until I experienced for myself the effects of sleeping over a stressed energy line.

Energy radiated upward from the earth is normally positive, but it can be distorted by underground water currents, mineral deposits, electric pylons and geological fractures, which cause the earth's electrical fields to radiate at unnaturally high frequencies. These distortions, called geopathic stress, can cause severe problems to anyone living, and particularly sleeping, over them.

The effects of geopathic stress include insomnia, depression, stress, respiratory problems and depletion of the immune system. It has been found to have a strong relationship with the development of cancer and other serious illnesses like Multiple Sclerosis: sometimes you come across a house in which whoever lives there develops a serious illness. Geopathic stress can also be the reason why some people never feel really well, while others don't recover from illness, whatever treatments they try.

In West Germany the problem is considered important enough for the government to have funded in 1987 a 400,000 DM research project to investigate the claim that cancer can be caused or exacerbated by living in an area of geopathic stress. And according to research in both Germany and Britain, there appears to be an important link between geopathic stress and cot death, the theory being that it weakens babies by affecting their immune system.

Geopathic stress may not actually *cause* cancer, depression and so on; what it appears to do is to trigger an illness towards which the person is already prone, or to magnify minor feelings of anxiety or depression. In my own case it is possible that the stress was caused by a re-routing of local water pipes, since I slept in the same room for many years before developing the symptoms of geopathic stress. I was recovering extremely slowly from a back problem, and at the same time found myself waking in the morning with extremely unpleasant and powerful sensations of anxiety, depression, and general horribleness. I had no way of knowing that what was probably a mild attack of self-doubt had been magnified a hundredfold, and began to wonder whether I was a candidate for psychiatry.

The cause was eventually pinpointed by a homoeopathic doctor whose wife confirmed the presence of geopathic stress through dowsing — for which I am eternally grateful. What was really convincing was that once the stress had been dealt with, I returned within a day or two, (and with enormous relief) to a normal state of mind. The experience has convinced me that geopathic stress is a very real and serious factor in our health, particularly in view of its possible connection with cot death.

It is hard to say how widespread this problem is. Dr Julian Kenyon, Director of the Centre for the Study of Complementary Medicine in Southampton, originally trained in orthodox medicine and now specializing in acupuncture, homoeopathy and research into the human energy fields, told me that geopathic stress is common enough to be considered seriously in insomniacs who don't respond to the normal methods.

Using a Vegatest (a diagnostic machine used by some doctors and natural practitioners) he finds that about 15-20 per cent of his patients suffer from geopathic stress; as he says, they are a highly selective population, but could still represent quite a lot of people.

The presence of geopathic stress is obviously of great importance to our physical and emotional health, and that of babies and children. How can you tell it's there?

The signs of geopathic stress

According to Dr Kenyon* and other experts like Rolf Gordon of the Dulwich Health Society (who believes his son would not have died of cancer if he had known about geopathic stress) these are some of the symptoms: insomnia, teeth-grinding, cramp, feeling cold in bed, sleep walking, restless sleep, depression on waking, exhaustion, and rheumatic aches and pains. There may obviously be other causes for all of these, but you might consider the presence of geopathic stress if:

You are not responding to treatments like homoeopathy and acupuncture.

Your cat regularly seeks out a specific spot to lie on. Most plants and animals will not thrive in geopathically stressed areas; for some curious reason they are favoured by ants, wasps, beetles, termites and cats (many young cats concurrently fall ill with leukaemia).

A sensitive person feels there is a bad atmosphere in the room.

A baby healthy at birth becomes weak within a few days for no other apparent reason.

A baby or small child sleeps restlessly and/or regularly moves to one side or the bottom of his or her bed or cot in an attempt to escape the harmful radiation.

An older child wets the bed, or suffers from nightmares.

Getting help

Geopathic stress can be diagnosed with the Vegatest machine mentioned above, if your practitioner has one. It can also be detected and dealt with by an experienced dowser, using dowsing rods on site, or a pendulum over a plan of your home. You may also be able to dowse for it yourself; instruction is included in Rolf Gordon's book *Are You Sleeping in a Safe Place?*†. Some good psychics and healers can also detect its presence and deal with it.

*Dr Julian Kenyon, 'Geopathic Stress', *Noma News*, (July 1989)
†See further reading at end of chapter

To contact a dowser in your area, write enclosing s.a.e. to The British Society of Dowsers, Sycamore Cottage, Tamley Lane, Hastingleigh, Ashford, Kent. The Society also runs courses in dowsing.

If geopathic stress is confirmed or suspected, dowsers have a variety of methods of counteracting it. For self-help, the most obvious solution is to move your bed to a non-affected place, which can also be found by dowsing. If this presents problems, temporary measures are to cover the floor under your bed with microwave cooking bags, which effectively block harmful radiation. Other blockers include cork matting under the bed or polythene sheeting between your mattress and the bottom sheet. However, cork matting eventually becomes saturated and will start radiating anew; and if the radiation is merely blocked it will reflect onto walls, or to the room below.

More permanent ways of dealing with it include the Raditech, a machine which counteracts harmful radiation as well as emitting negative ions. It plugs into an electric socket, and should be removed at intervals. It is available from the Dulwich Health Society, 130 Gipsy Hill, London SE19 1PL, tel. 081 670 5883, who will also confirm whether you are suffering from geopathic stress.

Crystals, particularly quartz or a combination of amethyst and pyrites, will absorb harmful radiations. They must be washed every day under cold running water.

Because there are different types of geopathic stress some methods work better in some cases than others; so whichever you try, you should retest the room after a month or so. You should also note that some people suffer from withdrawal symptoms for a while once the stress itself has been eradicated.

Further reading

Kathe Bachler, *Earth Radiation*, (available by mail order from Ilse Pope, 1 Garry Close, Romford, Essex RM1 4AE, tel. 0708 763809)

Roger Coghill, *Electropollution*, (Thorsons, 1990)

Rolf Gordon, *Are You Sleeping in a Safe Place?*, 1989, (available from The Dulwich Health Society, 130 Gipsy Hill, London SE19 1PL. Tel. 081 670 5883)

Cyril W. Smith & Simon Best, *Electromagnetic Man: Health and Hazard in the Electrical Environment*, (Dent, 1989)

PART 3

Towards good sleep

CHAPTER 1

Balancing your lifestyle

If you've read this far, you will probably have identified the causes of your insomnia, and some possible solutions. In this part of the book we'll be looking at ways for making your daytime life more conducive to night-time sleep. It's often said that it takes three weeks to change a habit. How long it will take you to break your habit of not sleeping I can't say — it may be sooner than you think. But three weeks is a good length of time to get yourself into a new rhythm of life and adopt habits which will help you towards acquiring a new, healthy sleep pattern.

Firstly, here's a check-list of some of the ground covered so far:

- Get a physical check-up if it seems appropriate.
- Stop thinking of yourself as insomniac, and start seeing yourself as well on the way to good sleep.
- Get up at the same time every day; don't nap during the day, or take lie-ins. Go to bed only when you feel sleepy.
- Notice how you talk to yourself, and start rebuilding your beliefs about both your sleep and yourself.
- Practise letting go of feelings that keep you awake, like anger and resentment, helping yourself with mental imagery.
- If you have unresolved problems, make a commitment during the next three weeks to finish unfinished business by taking action *during the day*, including getting help if you need it.

In this part of the book we'll be looking in more detail at further ways of helping yourself, including:

- Creating more fulfilment in your life.
- Getting regular non-competitive exercise appropriate to your needs and age.
- Learning to relax or meditate, and to include some relaxation

time in your daytime as well as night-time routine.
- Making sure you have a healthy diet geared to sleeping well.
- Winding down in the evenings and preparing yourself for peaceful sleep.

Start by taking an objective look at your life now, in order to draw yourself up a new programme. Insomniacs, as we've seen, fall broadly into four categories, which often overlap: the anxious and stressed, the depressed, the dissatisfied, and the angry. In all these groups there is a lack of balance, in that parts of yourself are dissatisfied, rumbling away in the background, and keeping you awake.

Now's the time to start filling in the gaps. If you never take time to relax, exercise, or play, now's the time to incorporate these activities into your programme. Only you know what your needs are: if you are very depressed or lethargic, at this point exercise may be more indicated than relaxation. Conversely, if you're a rusher-round, a regular daily period of relaxation or meditation may well be what you need. The idea is to balance up those parts of your life and of yourself that are currently being either over-used, or neglected, and to be nice to yourself.

A word of caution: if you're a perfectionist or over-stressed, don't stress yourself further by setting yourself impossible targets. Decide on the most important changes to make, and make them. As your physical and mental energies begin to flow, further change will follow naturally.

You may need to change your eating and other habits; if beating insomnia is really important to you, regard making these changes as an adventure rather than an imposition. The important thing is to know that you are now tackling your problems, and doing what's best for you.

Being kind to yourself

Perhaps most importantly of all, now's the time to start treating yourself kindly. We're often told how important it is to love ourselves; many insomniacs, it seems, suffer from low self-esteem. If you've never felt really loved or valued, 'loving yourself' can seem like a tall order — or perhaps like a pat answer without much real meaning. What it involves is simply respecting and valuing yourself as highly as you would any other human being, and behaving accordingly.

Loving yourself is yet another habit that can be cultivated. It may take time, and you may need help, perhaps by joining a therapy or assertiveness group. Meanwhile, simply start by treating yourself as kindly as you would like others to treat you.

If you have negative feelings towards yourself, they may well have been implanted there when you were a child. Imagine that you are now given the care of that child: talk to it lovingly, and appreciate all the good things about it. When you hear the voice of that inner critic in your head, tell it firmly that that is an old programme you no longer need.

Getting into the driving seat

Whatever the cause of your insomnia, if you want to sleep better at night, it's time to get into the driving seat and decide where you really want to go. What's missing from your life that would give you some real joy or peace of mind? Whatever it is needs to provide a contrast with your daily routine, not *more* of the same.

If you're a rusher-round, make time to do something totally unconnected with work. Do you do anything creative? Could you spend more time with your family — or less, if you're constantly fulfilling their needs? Are you really doing what you want to do, or have you some unfulfilled dream that your busy lifestyle, or those inner voices, have so far prevented you from achieving? If so, what first step can you take towards it?

If you're the unadventurous type, what could you do over this three-week period that would be a real challenge? Write a list of possibilities, things you've maybe thought of doing — if you only had the confidence. (They could include signing on at a self-assertion class.)

I'm not suggesting that you instantly chuck your job and family and go off to paint in Tahiti, like Gauguin. But we sometimes deny ourselves what we really want by telling ourselves it's impossible. Or we find perfectly reasonable excuses for not getting it, either because the idea of change is threatening, or we've simply got into the habit of self-denial.

Write a list of things you haven't done but would like to do. Be as fantastic as you like — if a journey to the moon comes to mind, write it down. At this stage, simply allow the ideas to flow, and if a critical inner voice jumps in to tell you not to be so silly, thank it and tell it it's your life, and you're in charge.

When you've written everything you can think of, look at that list as if it had been written by another person whom you are helping. What is really possible? Maybe it's too late to become a prima donna or ballerina: but perhaps you could join a singing or dancing class (either of which would help you to sleep by using your energy in a healthy way). You want to write a novel, but feel you're not talented enough? You'll never know until you've written it. You'd like a more exciting social life, but you never get any invitations? Remember, you're in the driving seat: take the first step and ask round the people you'd like to see more of.

Rushers-round may need less activity in their schedule, not more. You may be so strongly conditioned towards constant *doing* that 'doing nothing' doesn't appear on your list; it may actually be quite scary. Yet 'doing nothing', allowing yourself a little space, to think, to day-dream, to enjoy a walk in nature, may be just what's missing.

If you are depressed, it is really important to start moving, whether your depression is due to those inner voices, or to outer circumstances. If it's caused by unhappy life events like bereavement, redundancy, or divorce, it's a natural response. It's true that you do need to go through the grieving process before you feel fully yourself again; this can be true after a relationship breaks up just as much as following a death. But don't allow it to go on forever. Some people seem to stay stuck in their grief. If this is your case, it's important to take action to move yourself out of the slough of despond: to leave the unhappy past behind and take on new ventures — a new job, or voluntary work, a new hobby, or any interest that will move you forward and open up new horizons.

Perhaps your depression is due to life circumstances, such as unemployment, or the loneliness of being a single mother with small children. Don't let depression hold you back from helping yourself. Write down the aspects of your life that are making you unhappy. What can be changed? Can you get together with other people in the same boat to support each other, or join a self-help group? Make some kind of move, however small.

Perhaps you are depressed simply because you're depressed:

you don't like or love yourself much. Make a point of *behaving* as if you do. Depressed people often skip meals and don't bother about looking after their surroundings. A good start to defeating your negative inner voices is to look after yourself: include in your new programme a commitment to preparing proper meals and eating them slowly. Invite yourself to a particularly nice meal once a week; give yourself treats. Keep your bedroom and bedlinen tidy, fresh and clean, as if for a valued guest.

As I've said earlier, sometimes it's necessary to get help. It is not a sign of weakness to see a counsellor or psychotherapist. You've only got to listen to the radio phone-ins to agony aunts and uncles to realize that you're not alone in needing help — and also, how helpful even a few minutes with a professional can be. Maybe getting help could be included on your list.

Playtime

Most of our activities have a secondary purpose: to earn a living or keep the family and household going. One of the greatest pleasures of creative activities is doing them simply for their own sake, because you enjoy them.

An awful lot of our spare-time entertainment consists of watching other people do things, on television, at the cinema or sports matches. How much time do you spend actually *doing* something really enjoyable? Most people have a creative side which doesn't always get a look in. Whether you're over-stressed or not stressed enough, there's probably a corner of your mind in which there's an unfulfilled wish — that you'd taken up music, or painting, or hang-gliding, or acquired a degree. But of course, now it's too late, and you're too busy, or too old . . . That unfulfilled part of you may be contributing towards keeping you awake.

You don't have to be brilliantly talented to enjoy singing with a choir, or the pleasure of putting colours on canvas. You don't have to be a genius to enjoy the stimulation and companionship of a creative writing class, or the fun of belonging to an amateur theatrical group. Maybe you feel you've never exercised your brain enough; don't forget the Open University, or studying for A-levels at an evening class or by correspondence.

Even if you don't think you're particularly clever or creative, or your domestic set-up makes it difficult to get out to classes, skills like knitting or crochet, which engage your mind and hands gently, can be very satisfying. Some people find doing jigsaw puzzles immensely soothing. Growing plants, acquiring a pet, joining a cookery class — there are all kinds of ways in which you can take your mind away from anxiety or loneliness or depression, and focus it on something that gives you pleasure.

This is something you can do all the time, incidentally. So often we move about the world abstractedly, ruminating about the past or the future and missing out on present pleasures. Make a point of noticing what gives you pleasure or lifts your spirits as you go through the day, however small: a child's smile, the colours of nature, the sight of a brilliantly coloured flower-stall — do you pass these things by, or do you take them in and allow them to nourish your spirit?

It's never too late

Older people are often depressed simply because they feel lonely and useless. Family and friends move away or die, and it can feel as though nobody cares. But that may just be because nobody knows you're there. You may have to make the first move, but do make it. Old age in itself doesn't have to mean mental deterioration. Make sure that you have a regular routine, giving yourself proper meals and whatever exercise you can.

You may be entitled to rights that you don't know about, like getting a telephone installed; contact your town hall and find out about your entitlements. Even if your body is slowing down, look for outside activities that can provide company and mental stimulation. Some local authorities operate 'Adopt a Granny' schemes, which have given a new lease of life to many elderly women who find themselves wanted members of a family again. Lots of families would appreciate baby-sitting services. Your local social services department or health visitor may be able to let you know of local groups that you can join.

It's never too late for further education. Many older people get a great deal of stimulation — and company — from adult education classes. There is also The University of the Third Age, which has a number of branches countrywide. Their head office is c/o BASSAC, 13 Stockwell Road, London SW9 9AU, tel. 071 737 2541.

Living in the present

Anxiety and sadness, anger and resentment, are always concerned with either past or future. If you are totally focused in the present moment you *can't* be anxious. So try to take opportunities of living in the present as much as you can.

Put your full attention on whatever you are doing at the time when you're doing it, whether it's working, walking, or washing up. Let your thinking mind off the hook for a few minutes; pause and be aware of your physical body, of your feet on the ground, and your surroundings. If you are out walking, simply look at and experience the sights and sounds, without getting involved in a long train of thought. Gradually you will learn to switch off that over-busy mind and give it and you a rest.

Happiness, the opposite of anxiety and depression, is only ever found in the present moment. We look back with nostalgia, thinking 'If only things had been different!', or forward to achievements we believe will make us feel good; or we believe that someone else could make us happy, if only they would behave differently.

If you remember the real moments of happiness in your life you will know that they don't really depend on other people or events, but on feeling good with yourself. Living in the present helps us to accept ourselves as we are, without judging ourselves by other people's standards. It takes practice, and may not come easily at first, but it's another habit that can be cultivated. And it's a healing habit: one woman totally cured her depression by living in the present, giving up all regrets about the past and fears for the future.

It's also a habit you can take to bed with you. Instead of worrying about whether or when you are going to get to sleep, simply be with yourself in the present moment, regretting nothing, expecting nothing, giving your body and mind permission to let go a d rest.

CHAPTER 2

A change of pace

Over the last few years the media have made it very clear that exercise is good for us. For the sake of your sleep you really do need to exercise regularly; the occasional burst won't do much for you. One experiment showed that a single bout of strenuous daytime exercise increased the amount of slow-wave sleep that night in people who were already fit, but had no effect on the sleep of the unfit. On the other hand, research shows that athletes who exercise consistently seem to have more deep, delta sleep than non-exercisers, and when deprived of their exercise their delta sleep diminishes.

If you are physically unable to exercise, don't despair. According to Dr James Horne, there is no fall in slow-wave sleep in paraplegics or people obliged to take long periods of bed-rest.*
It seems as if the body-mind system adjusts to such situations. But the potentially active body, under-used, will express its dissatisfaction by keeping you awake.

Regular exercise undoubtedly contributes to general health and well-being. For one thing, it tires the body in a healthy way — which is quite different from the tiredness you feel when you've been rushing round getting mentally exhausted, or not rushing round, and getting bored and frustrated.

Exercise is also a wonderful way of clearing the body of the stress hormones that keep so many people awake, anxious or depressed. It can also help to clear your body if you are giving up smoking, alcohol or any other kind of drug. It's also a wonderful way to get over depression or grief. Some people have lifted themselves right out of depression through regular

*James Horne, *Why We Sleep*, (Oxford University Press, 1988)

running or jogging. And a widowed friend of mine coped with the worst of her bereavement by joining a rambling club and walking for miles every weekend — an excellent recipe for good sleep.

A word of caution: avoid taking exercise late at night, which actually over-stimulates the body. One man who sought help for insomnia was found to be running for several miles late every night. The simple answer was to schedule his exercise earlier in the day. For sleeping purposes, while a gentle walk round the block to unwind last thing is fine, the best times for strenuous exercise are the afternoon and early evening.

What kind of exercise?

If you're out of training, don't go in for a sudden enthusiastic burst and then give up on it; build up slowly and naturally. Try walking rather than driving or taking public transport to the station or to work; climb stairs rather than taking lifts. If you normally spend your lunch hour in a pub or canteen, try to take twenty to thirty minutes of that time walking (and I don't mean shopping).

If you're not geared to exercising, it really is very helpful to join a class; having a regular commitment to a group helps to keep you motivated. It's also a good way of making new friends. Have a look at what's available at your local evening institute, adult education or health centre. Competitive sports like tennis, squash and golf can also be beneficial, but not if losing makes you upset or angry. Games are supposed to be enjoyable.

If you're a rusher-round consider taking up a calming form of movement, like T'ai Chi or Yoga. Both will help to balance your energy system, as well as calming mind and body, and both can help you to face life with more tranquillity. Swimming is good, too, with its rhythmic movement and deep breathing; so is walking in the country.

If you are anxious or depressed pick a class with plenty of movement — again, make sure it's enjoyable, not a form of self-punishment. Aerobics, modern and jazz dance, and Medau movement are all cheering and energizing. Any kind of dance is good; some women who've taken up Spanish or Egyptian dancing have found a side benefit in the form of greater self-esteem. Even bopping to the radio or a tape at home can quickly lift your spirits; it's really difficult to be depressed when you're dancing.

For self-esteem, the increasingly popular martial arts are also good. Aikido or judo, for instance, will strengthen both your body and your sense of yourself.

If you are retired getting enough exercise will help to keep you healthy and youthful. If you've let yourself go, build up slowly, but add a bit more movement to your day, even if it's just an extra walk round the block. Evening institutes often arrange movement and even yoga classes of the over 60s.

Whatever type you decide on, commit yourself to exercising regularly; build up slowly, and enjoy it.

Relaxation and meditation

The onset of normal sleep is a drowsy, relaxed state, a state of peaceful letting go. It should be a state that we drift into naturally, yet in this busy, stressed age, many people have simply lost the art of relaxation, and have to relearn it.

Watching television, going to the cinema, socializing and other off-duty activities all have their place, but they are not really relaxing.

True relaxation involves switching off the active right brain, and also the part of the nervous system that gears us up for action. It reverses the process of building up tension by bringing into play the parasympathetic nervous system, which counteracts the effects of stress, and helps to strengthen the immune system. Regular relaxation can actually alter body chemistry, and deep states can help the brain to produce endorphins, hormones that have been called 'the body's own morphine', which have the effects of lifting the mood and relieving pain.

Meditation has many similar effects. Though relaxation is aimed chiefly at the body, and meditation at the mind and spirit, both slow down and rebalance the body-mind system. Many people who meditate regularly find they need less sleep than before, because during their meditation periods they are giving their systems deep rest. Both meditation and relaxation require us, and also enable us, to let go of worry and tension and focus on the present moment.

Some people are quite scared of letting go; they feel they must hang on and stay in control. This is partly because many of us have been brought up with the idea that 'doing nothing' is a waste of precious time, possibly even sinful; partly because of a not always conscious fear that something terrible will happen if we let go. The most vivid example of this I ever saw was on a plane journey with a friend who was scared of flying: she sat rigid in her seat clutching the armrests, and I suddenly realized that *she was actually trying to hold the plane up.*

Letting go is a normal part of life's rhythm; hanging on to control builds up physical tensions which go to bed with you. A tense mind is less able to solve problems than a relaxed one: if you learn to relax you will find that it will not make you less efficient, but better able to cope, and with more control over your waking and sleeping patterns.

In 1985 a small study was carried out by the Sleep Laboratory at Leeds University, with a group of airline pilots. Pilots have such irregular hours and routines that they often have to take sleeping pills to get their rest, a far from ideal situation. Ten pilots were taught a mixture of muscle relaxation and mental meditational techniques, which enabled them to get to sleep whenever they needed to, in unusual environments, even on long taxi-rides. Eight months later, seven of them were still using these techniques; of the remaining three, one had been practising his own form of meditation before the study.

Most people in these tense days could benefit from regular relaxation or meditation. Build it into your day: give yourself a space to practise for 20 minutes at least once a day.

Learning to relax

Although there are some excellent books on relaxation I feel that if you are under severe tension, there is nothing to beat personal tuition, in a group or class where you can get individual attention.

If you want to make a start on your own, choose a time and a place where you will be peaceful and undisturbed. Tell yourself that you are going to devote the next 20 minutes to completely letting go. (The aeroplane won't fall down!) Sit comfortably with your back supported and your feet flat on the floor, your hands loose in your lap and your eyes closed. Or lie down, with your head and knees supported by cushions. There are several relaxation techniques favoured by experts. Here are two.

Progressive relaxation consists of alternately tensing and relaxing all the muscles in your body, from toe to head, or head to toe, in turn. Take it slowly. When you've been through all the muscles, notice if there are any tense spots left, and let them go. The jaw is often a tension-site; clench it and then let it drop. Make sure your tongue is relaxed too. Then enjoy the sense of relaxation until your 20 minutes are up. Come out of it slowly; if you jump up you may find yourself slightly giddy.

Another method is to start sitting or lying, stretch the whole body, and let it go, like a cat. Then simply sense that waves of relaxation are flowing through your body as you breathe in, while more and more tension is leaving you with every out-breath.

Relaxation can be aided by using mental imagery: as you let go physically, imagine that you are floating on a cloud or on a lilo on a sun-lit sea; or that you are a cat, totally relaxed and oblivious of your surroundings; or a heavy sackful of sand; or a balloon floating in a blue sky. (Images of both lightness and heaviness seem to aid relaxation equally well.)

Cassette tapes can also help you learn to relax on your own; there are a number of good ones on the market. Don't, however, become dependent on one tape. What you are aiming for is the ability to relax whenever you want to — not just at special relaxation times.

Meditation techniques

These take you into a relaxed state through the mind. Their object is to reach a state of inner peace by quietening mental chatter, often by focusing on a word, sound, or object. Again, I feel it's important that meditation should be taught personally or in a group; the inexperienced meditator often strains to concentrate, and guidance may be needed in letting go.

If you want to try it for yourself, start with five or ten minutes at a time. Sit as for the relaxation exercise above, making sure you won't be disturbed. Then try one of the following:

Gently repeat mentally a single word, for example 'harmony'.

Rest your attention on this word without straining. Every time you find your mind wandering, bring it back to the word.

Put your attention on your breathing, simply being aware of it without trying to change it. It can help you to concentrate if you count from one to ten as you do so, counting 'one-and', 'two-and' and so on with each in-out breath. If you lose count, return to one.

At the end of any relaxation or meditation exercise, don't leap back into activity, but come out slowly and gently, bringing some of that inner peace into the rest of your life.

Research shows that several relaxation techniques can be beneficial for insomniacs, including progressive relaxation, relaxation-meditation, biofeedback assisted meditation and autogenic training (described below). Whatever method is used, it needs to be practised regularly, both with an instructor and at home.*

Some people find it difficult to relax because they simply don't know what relaxation feels like. Many of the natural therapies can help you to regain that experience, particularly hands-on treatments like the Alexander Technique, massage, cranial osteopathy and spiritual healing. Some forms of exercise are also very relaxing; Yoga includes techniques for whole-body relaxation and meditation, while T'ai Chi has been described as meditation in movement.

Breathing

Correct breathing is important in both relaxation and meditation. As body and mind slow down, so does the breath; conversely, slowing and deepening your breathing automatically makes you calmer. However, when we are tense we tend to breathe fast and shallowly, high up in the chest, which makes it very hard to relax. Some chronically tense people hyperventilate; that is, they over-breathe all the time, which keeps them in a permanent state of anxiety. Hyperventilation also prevents sufficient oxygen reaching the brain and can have other

*S.J.E. Lindsay, 'Disorders of Sleep: Treatment', *A Handbook of Clinical Adult Psychology*, Stan Lindsay and Graham Powell (eds.), (Gower Publishing, 1987)

unpleasant side effects like migraines, dizziness, nausea and palpitations.

Learning to breathe naturally helps you to keep calm. Try this: lie on the floor with a cushion or book under your head. Put a heavy-ish object (a large book or a beanbag) on your midriff, between your abdomen and lower ribs. As you breathe in and out, the object should rise and fall; if it doesn't, you are breathing too high up in the chest.

Using the weight as a guide, you can retrain yourself to breathe diaphragmatically: full breathing should expand your diaphragm, lower ribs, and abdomen. Don't *force* yourself to breathe deeply; simply be aware of how you are breathing now. Then think of your ribs and lungs expanding and contracting, and allow your breath to become deeper, slower and calmer. Think of your ribs expanding sideways as well as up and down. If you practise this for a few minutes every day, you will acquire the habit of calmer, relaxing breathing when you get to bed at night.

Another sign of anxiety is holding your breath. A good exercise when you feel yourself tensing up during the day is to consciously breathe out, at the same time letting the tension flow away from your neck, shoulders and arms. Practise this in situations which would normally make you uptight: in traffic jams and queues, or waiting to be put through on the telephone. As it starts to become a habitual response, you can use these occasions as opportunities for relaxation instead of anxiety, irritation or anger.

A good method of getting back in touch with your body and breathing pattern is the Alexander Technique, which (among its other benefits) helps to free tensions locked into the back and rib-cage. Osteopathy and chiropractic can also help to free tight chest muscles, enabling you to breathe more fully. Yoga, too, lays much stress on breathing; one very simple exercise is to breathe in to the count of six, hold your breath to the count of six, breathe out to the count of six, and then either breathe in again or hold the outbreath for six, before resuming the cycle. It is very calming.

Relaxation and pain

Relaxation is one of the techniques employed in pain relief clinics, and research into its benefits has been carried out in London hospitals. Properly taught, it has been found to reduce not only anxiety but the amount of painkillers required after operations.

There are two possible ways of dealing with pain: to accept it and relax into it, or to focus your mind on something completely different. Although these two methods might seem contradictory, what they have in common is that both remove the *resistance* to pain. Resisting pain always makes it worse; tensing up against it tightens muscles and restricts the flow of blood. Mentally resisting also makes it worse. So, some alternatives are:

Learn to relax *into* the pain, accepting it as a bodily sensation without labelling it 'pain' or wondering if it's ever going to stop. Breathing into the site of the pain is also helpful, letting go of the pain as you breathe out.

Use imagery while you relax, perhaps visualizing the pain as a blob of colour which slowly melts, running out of the body through your fingers or toes.

Focus on something other than the pain, so long as it's something pleasant: imagine yourself in beautiful surroundings, or remember a place where you have felt particularly happy and peaceful.

Aids to learning to relax

(Enclose s.a.e. with written enquiries.)

Autogenic training is an eight-week course in learning to relax body and mind very deeply; it verges on meditation, and uses imagery as well as physical techniques. Techniques are also taught for releasing emotions like anger and fear. Because it can bring about deep physical change it is only taught by people with medical training. Details of trainers from:
The Positive Health Centre,
101 Harley Street,
London W1N 1DF
Tel. 071 935 1822.

Biodfeedback training can be extremely helpful in teaching people to relax at will, and biodfeedback therapists use ·a combination of relaxation and meditational techniques. Various instruments are used to measure and help you recognize your states of mental and physical tension and relaxation, so that you learn to produce a more relaxed state at will. There are a few biofeedback clinics in hospitals (ask your GP). For private classes, practitioners and courses, contact:
Audio Ltd,
26-28 Wendell Road,
London W12 9RT
Tel. 081 743 1518/4352

Hypnotherapy relaxes both body and mind. (See Part 1, Chapter 3.)

Relaxation for Living will provide details of teachers and classes throughout the country; they also have tapes available for sleep problems and other stress-related disorders. Send a large s.a.e. to:
29 Burwood Park Road,
Walton-on-Thames,
Surrey KT12 5LH
Tel. 093 22 27826

Further reading

Herbert Benson MD, *The Relaxation Response*, (Collins Fountain Books, 1977)

Ursula Fleming, *Grasping the Nettle; A Positive Approach to Pain*, (Collins Fountain Books, 1990). The author has also made a series of relaxation tapes, including *Relax to Ease Pain* and *Relax to Ease Stress*; details from: Ursula Fleming Tapes, PO Box 1902, London NW3 2UF.

Lawrence LeShan, *How to Meditate: A Guide to Self-Discovery*, (Crucible, 1989)

Jane Madders, *Stress and Relaxation*, (Martin Dunitz, 1979)

CHAPTER 3

Food and other habits

It's impossible to get a really healthy balance in life without including nutrition. Food and drink have a direct chemical influence on our bodies, nervous system and moods. Over-indulgence in junk food, coffee or alcohol — all of which often accompany a stressed lifestyle — affects your well-being, simultaneously over-stimulating the adrenal glands and nervous system and depleting the body of essential vitamins and minerals. In addition, some foods are more stimulating and some more sedative in their own right.

We get many contradictory messages these days about what's good for us and what isn't. And of course individual needs differ; while more and more people are becoming vegetarian, for instance, there are others whose systems really seem to need meat. If you're in any doubt, consult a naturopath or nutritionist about your needs. Meanwhile, here are some general guidelines which hold good for everyone who wants to sleep better.

Foods and drinks to go for:

Plenty of fresh fruit and salads, dried fruits, green and root vegetables, *live* yoghurt (if it suits you), whole grains (brown rice, oats, wholemeal bread and flour), pulses (lentils and dried beans), fish and free-range chicken rather than red meats, and a moderate amount of fats, eggs, cheese and dairy products. Among these foods, the more stimulating are raw vegetables, salads and fruits; so naturopaths recommend fruit and/or dried fruit with breakfast and a large raw salad with lunch.

Root vegetables are believed to be more sedative than those growing above ground; also sedative are the unrefined carbo-hydrates — potatoes, and wholegrain bread, pasta and rice, so these are best eaten with the evening meal.

Many foods, when combined with carbohydrates, lead to the production of an amino-acid called tryptophan, the main building block for serotonin, a neurochemical which is produced as a precursor to sleep. They include milk, eggs, meat, nuts, fish, hard cheeses, bananas and pulses.*

Drink herbal teas, spring water and pure fruit juices, or some of the non-caffeinated drinks you can buy in health food stores, such as dandelion coffee (made from the dried root rather than powder), or cereal drinks like Barley Cup and Pionier.

Food and drinks to avoid:

Sugar (including cakes, chocolate, biscuits etc.)

Refined carbohydrates (white flour and sugar), which fill you up and overwork the digestive system without giving your body any real fuel.

Processed foods. We have been made aware of the dangers of chemical additives, especially to the allergy-prone, but many processed foods still contain additives to which some people have an adverse reaction without always realizing it. In particular, tartrazine (E102) and monosodium glutamate can upset people's sleeping patterns, especially if eaten in the evening.

High-fat foods also put a strain on the digestive system when eaten in the evening — so there may be some truth in the suggestion that cheese can give you bad dreams!

Caffeine, found not just in coffee, but in tea, colas, and chocolate, doesn't only affect you late at night. It can contribute to nervousness and depression at any time.

Excess salt raises the blood pressure and puts the body into overdrive.

---

*In the 1980s a supplement called L-tryptophan was promoted as a natural answer to sleeplessness. Alas, scientists are still looking for that 'natural' sleeping pill, for in 1989 L-tryptophan fell under suspicion when a number of American consumers of these supplements fell ill with a serious flu-like disease. No bad affects have been reported in the UK, and the problem may have been caused by contamination of imported batches. However, early in 1990, scientists had not discounted the possibility that the supplement itself was causing the problem.

The timing of meals

Far less well publicized than what we eat is the importance of *when* we eat. The old adage, 'breakfast like a king, lunch like a lord and dine like a pauper', is supported by naturopaths and other natural practitioners, who recommend a hearty breakfast, a moderate lunch, and a light supper, eaten if possible no later than 6 p.m.

There are very good biological reasons for this: the human digestive system functions best in the morning, when it produces a good supply of enzymes for the quick and efficient absorption of nutrients. The digestive process gets slower throughout the day, really starting to slow down around 6 p.m.; by nine it is very sluggish indeed.

You may *feel* sleepy after a heavy meal, because the blood goes from the head to the stomach, but still find it difficult to get to sleep because your body has been given an extra hard task when it should be resting — *you* wouldn't like to start work at bedtime either! In addition, digestion takes place most efficiently when the body is upright.

Although people's body clocks differ, the slowing down of digestion seems to be true for everyone. This means that food eaten late in the evening is liable to remain in the stomach half-digested and putrefying all night, affecting both sleep and our enthusiasm for breakfast in the morning. In some cases it can actually cause a build-up of toxins, leading to ill-health.

If you habitually sleep badly, a large breakfast may well be the last thing you feel like in the morning. But remember that you are now changing your habits to encourage your body to relax and sleep; how you start the day will affect how you end it. If you try for a three-week period having a good lunch and an early, light supper, you'll soon find yourself much keener on breakfast.

A hearty and healthy breakfast could include porridge, or an oat-based muesli (oats are excellent nerve strengtheners) with yoghurt and dried or fresh fruit, and/or wholemeal toast with honey, or cheese if you like it. No more than three eggs (preferably free-range) should be eaten per week.

Unfortunately, our social system is not geared to our body clocks and for the rest of the day you may have to do some adaptation. The lordly lunch accompanied by a large salad may not be available where you work, and if you have a long journey home, the early, light supper may present difficulties. Experiment with packed lunches; raw carrots, celery and apples need scarcely any preparation. If possible, finish your evening meal by 8 p.m. at the latest.

If you are going straight from work to an evening class, have your hot meal at lunchtime and a sandwich or baked potato before the class. And if you're invited out for a late, delicious dinner — keep the portions down (and the alcohol), relax and enjoy it! Eating *happily* is possibly as important as what you eat.

Some therapists believe the timing of meals is all-important. Practitioners of Reconnective Therapy (see Part 4), recommend a regime called 'the Way of Life'. This involves rising early (at 5 or 6 a.m.) to eat your main meal before 9 a.m., when food is most efficiently transformed into energy. At this time, you can eat virtually anything you like; you can do much of the preparation the evening before. Meals should be accompanied by plenty of fluid. Lunch, one third the size of breakfast, should be finished by 2 p.m. — and that's it for the day. You then go to bed at 9 p.m. five nights a week, on the basis that the most restorative sleep is before midnight.

Extreme as this system may sound, many people who have tried it find that they have more energy, and feel happier and more positive generally. Following the Way of Life enables you to have your cake and eat it: you can enjoy the foods you like in the morning, and give yourself a mini-fast every evening, resting your digestion, and detoxifying and normalizing your body.

By balancing your system, and working in co-operation with your body clock, the Way of Life can be a very good way to combat insomnia. Some people have to overcome a certain amount of resistance to making such a big change in their habits; others find it suits their lifestyle and take to it like ducks to water.

Allergies and sensitivities

If you suffer severely from a food allergy you will probably already be aware of it. But degrees of allergic reaction vary; some people are sensitive to particular foods without having an out-and-out allergy. Their degree of sensitivity can also vary, with reactions worse at particularly stressful times and unnoticeable at others. The substances most commonly causing allergic reactions or intolerance are wheat, eggs, dairy products, sugar and caffeine, as well as certain chemicals and additives.

Very often, people are unaware that something they've been enjoying for years is affecting them badly. This is a common phenomenon known as a masked allergy, when sufferers are actually addicted to the substance that is doing them harm.

It's worth observing your reactions to foods and drinks, particularly those you crave for or consume every day. If you notice that you regularly feel extra hyped up or depressed after any of these, try cutting them out of your diet for a week or two and see whether this makes a difference. If you are suffering from a masked allergy you may get slight withdrawal symptoms; people giving up caffeine, for instance, sometimes experience headaches and fuzziness for a few days. If this happens to you, tell yourself it's actually a good sign, showing that your system is cleansing itself of something that was doing it harm. Drink plenty of spring water to help it along.

Supplements

Views on the value of vitamin and mineral supplements vary wildly, particularly between orthodox medical doctors and supplement-minded practitioners. The general orthodox view is that so long long as you eat a healthy, balanced diet, you don't need anything extra. However, natural therapists point out that so much of our food is de-natured by things like pesticides, pollution and preservatives that most people's vitamin and mineral intake needs topping up. This is certainly so when someone is under stress, as is likely to be the case with insomniacs.

At the same time, supplements are only useful when they supply what you personally are short of. Taking more of a vitamin or mineral than you actually need is wasteful, and can in some cases be harmful; in others, taking supplements will have no effect if for some reason your body is not absorbing them. On top of this, there is an increasingly bewildering array in health food shops of not only vitamins and herbal remedies but amino-acids and unusual minerals. Advice from a homoeopath, naturopath, nutritionist, or kinesiologist (see Part 4) can help you to sort out your personal needs, and may save you a lot of expense on unnecessary, useless, or incompletely researched supplements.

In general, however, it can be both helpful and safe to take a good combined vitamin and mineral pill daily. If you are highly stressed you can safely take daily an extra 1000mg of Vitamin C (with bioflavonoids) and 25mg B6 (which helps the body make use of tryptophan); this should be accompanied by a B-complex tablet. If you smoke, you need extra amounts of both B and C since nicotine leaches these vitamins, as well as some minerals, from the system.

The mineral calcium is widely recommended for nerves and anxiety; a naturopath recommends taking 200mg daily in the form of Dolomite tablets, which contain natural calcium combined with magnesium, another stress reducer which also helps the body to absorb the calcium. Zinc can also be useful, particularly if you are depressed; since this comes in many varieties, consult your health food shop owner or natural health practitioner before buying.

A word about alcohol

It's true that a small amount of alcohol is a relaxant, and can blur the edges of anxiety. But there are both disadvantages and risks in the alcoholic night-cap. Alcohol is a drug: it's possible for one glass to turn into two, or more . . . and before you know it you have developed a dependency. And even if it helps you to get off to sleep initially, alcohol can actually *cause* insomnia. To digest it, your liver and kidneys have to work extra hard, and your body has to provide extra adrenalin — which is, of course, a stimulant. It has been found that after alcohol intake, sleep is more disturbed with more awakenings; alcohol also reduces REM sleep.

Drinking large amounts of alcohol regularly can lead to alcohol addiction — alcoholism, in other words — which affects your body, your work, and your relationships, and your sleep.

So, ideally, stick to no more than a glass or two of wine, two or three days a week; you'll feel better for it all round. If you feel deprived on non-alcohol days, boost your morale by telling yourself you're giving your body — especially your hard-working liver — a nice rest!

If you find it really difficult to have a non-alcohol day, it could be that you have a real problem. Alcohol addiction is something that people find it very hard to admit to; as an AA member once said to me, 'It's the one disease that tells you you haven't got it!' But if you really want to lead a more balanced life, and suspect you may be addicted, it is vital to acknowledge the fact and deal with it. It is not something to be ashamed of. Drinking is a socially acceptable way of coping with stress; unfortunately it can create further stress. There are healthier options.

You will find a local branch of Alcoholics Anonymous in your phone book; don't be embarrassed to get in touch with them for a talk. They are nice, helpful people, who recognize alcoholism as a disease rather than a character defect. There are also organizations which use counselling and group therapy to help people cut down on their alcohol intake without giving up altogether. These include Accept (200 Seagrave Road, London SW6 1RQ, tel. 071 381 3155). Consult your doctor, or contact your local Citizens Advice Bureau for details of local organizations who can help.

Smoking

Nicotine is also a stimulant, which can exacerbate sleepless-ness, particularly as you grow older. Non-insomniac smokers have been found to take longer to go to sleep than non-smokers and wake up more often during the night. In a trial at Penn-sylvania State University, when eight heavy smokers gave up abruptly, the time they took to get to sleep dropped from an average 52 minutes to 18 on the first two nights, and this pattern continued in four of them who continued without smoking for two weeks.

Initially, giving up may cause a short-term increase in tension, and if you are under a lot of stress at the moment this may not be the best time to stop. But do cut down, especially in the evenings, and try not to smoke during the last hour before going to bed. One way of cutting down is to tell yourself, every time you reach for a cigarette, that you'll have it later.

If you make a real commitment to stop, this could obviously improve your sleep quite rapidly. You can get many forms of help and support from a number of natural therapies which will help to calm your nervous system and support you during the withdrawal phase. These include a choice of acupuncture, homoeopathy, herbalism, hypnotherapy, kinesiology, and relaxation.

Further information

(Send s.a.e. with written enquiries)

For information about coping with allergies contact:
Action Against Allergy,
43 The Downs,
Wimbledon,
London SW20 8HG
Tel. 081 947 5082

Full details of the Way of Life are obtainable from:
Annick Labouré,
The Natural Reconnective Therapy School,
P.O. Box 630,
Hove,
E. Sussex BN3 6BQ

Further reading

Dr Jonathan Brostoff and Linda Gamlin, *The Complete Guide to Food Allergy and Intolerance*, (Bloomsbury Press, 1989)
Dr Stephen Davies and Dr Alan Stewart, *Nutritional Medicine*, (Pan, 1987)
Patrick Holford, *Vitamin Vitality*, (Collins, 1985)

CHAPTER 4

Bedtime

The hour or two leading up to bedtime should be a time of slowly winding-down, letting go of the day and its busyness. If you need to have a family discussion (or worse), get it over early, and leave matters as resolved as they can be. Write down anything unresolved, and make a definite appointment with yourself and anyone else involved to continue it another time, not in bed.

The same goes for anything else that might be worrying you. Early in the evening, write it down, write down any decisions you have made about dealing with it, and then say goodbye to it for today. *You have done all you can.*

Keep your bedtime as regular as possible; while you are retraining your body-mind system, late nights are not a good idea. Although scientifically it's not been proven that the hours before midnight are best for sleep, some natural practitioners believe that they are. Round about ten p.m. our body clocks begin to slow down and gear themselves for sleep.

Try to observe your own natural rhythm, and don't stay up beyond the time when you naturally feel sleepy, even if that means foregoing the end of an interesting TV programme. Some experts recommend that you don't watch television during the hour before bedtime, since the flickering image can stimulate the nervous system. However, I think this must depend on both the person and the programme. A cheering or funny programme may help you go to bed in a good mood. But don't fall asleep while you're watching it: you'll have to wake up again in order to go to bed — very confusing to your body clock, which then makes it hard to get off again.

The same goes for reading in bed. While the stimulus-control programme says the bedroom is only for sleep, some people do find reading in bed a good way to switch their mind away from the worries of the day. This again must be your own choice. But don't waver between systems: if you've chosen to adopt the stimulus-control programme, stick to it for the whole three weeks.

Bedtime drinks

A hot bedtime drink can be soothing and comforting — but bear in mind that it will reach your bladder in the small hours. This might seem obvious, but I've come across more than one elderly person complaining of having to get up to go to the bathroom, without connecting it with their late-night cup of tea! As we get older our kidneys become more active during the night, so the amount an elderly person can comfortably drink before bed will be less than in his or her younger days. If your bladder is a problem, try having your bedtime drink no later than an hour before bedtime.

The tradition of having a hot milky drink at bedtime is probably based on the fact that milk contains both tryptophan and calcium, which is a muscle relaxant and soothing to the nervous system. A cup of hot milk accompanied by a couple of Dolomite tablets (containing calcium and magnesium) can help you get off to sleep, and helps some sufferers from restless legs.

Not all proprietary milky drinks are actually good for sleep; chocolate, for instance, has a high caffeine content. Best is plain hot milk, with maybe a teaspoon of honey, or a malted milk like Horlicks. A sprinkling of grated nutmeg on top is also sleep inducing. If your sleeplessness is related to indigestion, Slippery Elm makes a soothing drink.

Some people find milk hard to digest, and as it is a food in its own right dietary purists would not recommend it last thing at night. This also applies to late night snacks, of course. Some people recommend eating a snack of foods containing trypto- phan last thing at night — a bowl of cereal, a banana, or a lettuce sandwich for instance. As discussed in the last chapter, this is the time when the body should be geared for sleep, not for digesting food — and food eaten last thing is more likely to end up as stored fat.

However, this is a choice you must make for yourself: if a late-night snack suits you and helps you sleep, that may be the most important factor while you recover your sleep pattern.

Some people find cider vinegar and honey helps them to sleep; the mixture contains a good supply of trace elements including calcium. Take a teaspoonful of each in a small cup of boiling water.

A very pleasant late-night drink is Norfolk Punch, a non-alcoholic blend of herbs and spices found in health food shops recommended as a relaxant. Some people find that it loses its efficacy if drunk every night; have it as a treat after a particularly fraught day.

Herbal drinks

Herb teas are becoming increasingly popular as replacements for caffeine-containing drinks. There is a good variety of herbal tea-bags in the shops, some of them specially blended to help you relax or sleep. They are quite expensive; it's cheaper to buy loose herbs from a herbalist or health food shop and experiment with single herbs or mixtures. Herbs can lose their efficacy over time, so buy them in small quantities, keep them in an air-tight jar, and use them promptly.

Herbal infusions

Herbal infusions are slightly stronger than teas, and can be taken medicinally three times a day. You can make up an infusion of one or more herbs, using 1-2 heaped teaspoonfuls of dried leaves or flowers to a cup of water. Use a herbal infuser or small teapot, and pour the water onto the herbs when just on the boil. Leave to stand, covered, for at least 5-10 minutes before drinking, up to 20 minutes if you are taking them medicinally.

Children and babies will respond to smaller doses; where an adult takes a cupful, a 10-year-old can have a small glass, a toddler a tablespoon and a baby small, occasional sips.

Camomile is one of the best-known herbs for calming the nerves, and for settling the digestion. It is said to have cumulative effects, becoming more effective over a period of time. However, some people find the flavour rather bland, and it has the disadvantage of being mildly diuretic.

Lime-flower (linden) makes a very effective and pleasant flavoured night-cap and is good for headaches, nervous tension and restlessness. The herbalist Michael McIntyre, co-author of *The Complete New Herbal** told me that when he lived in France hyperactive children would be taken out to have tea under the lime trees in summer, because of their calming effect. And it didn't only calm children. 'The bees were narcotized,' he said. 'You'd see them lying there glugging gently because they'd had a bit too much lime flower while taking the nectar!' (A nice image to go to bed with!)

Scullcap is a tonic as well as a sedative, high in magnesium and calcium, which help to strengthen the nervous system. It is not always easy to obtain, and what is often sold as scullcap is another herb called teucrium (wood sage). So get the genuine article, *Scutellaria laterifolia*, from a reputable herbalist.

Passiflora (passion flower) is another good soporific, a constituent of many herbal sleeping pills.

Valerian root is well-known as a sedative. It tastes like old socks (and smells worse) but a proportion of it can be mixed with more pleasant-flavoured herbs. Valerian has a more 'druggy' effect than most herbs, and some people find it gives them headaches if drunk in large quantities; so (unless prescribed by a herbalist) don't take it consecutively for more than a week or two.

Hawthorn flowers are good for people who don't sleep because they have heart palpitations.

Mint is good for soothing the digestion.

Lemon Balm and vervain are good for depression.

Bath-time

Wash off any remaining stresses of the day by having a bath before bed, and make it sleep inducing with the help of herbal or aromatherapy preparations. Enjoy your bath as a relaxing treatment; make it warm but not too hot, and give yourself time to soak in the oils or herbs so that you get the full, soothing benefit.

Suitable aromatherapy oils include lavender (used regularly it

*Richard Mabey (ed.), *The Complete New Herbal*, (Elm Tree Books, 1988)

has the advantage of boosting your immune system, but go easy on it if you are pregnant), camomile and orange blossom (both rather expensive), meadowsweet, geranium and hops. Use no more than four to six drops of oil or oils altogether, using the smaller amount if your skin is very sensitive. Agitate the water so that the oil spreads evenly and reaches your whole body. Allow yourself time to soak, relax and absorb the oil both through your skin and by inhaling the vapour.

Herbs can also be used in the bath by making an extra strong infusion, steeped, strained and poured into your bath water. Lime-flowers are good; so are hops: pour a cup of boiling water over three crushed heads and steep, covered, for ten minutes. You can also use lavender, or a mixture of herbs: fill a muslin bag with the heads and tie it to the hot tap, so that the hot water runs through it. Before getting into the bath, add a strained infusion of the same herbs.

Herbal baths are also soothing for babies. Michael McIntyre says: 'Camomile herb is a very suitable way to get your baby to sleep. You can give your baby a camomile bath. Make a strong tea using an ounce to two pints of water, strain it, and add it to the water in the baby-bath.' And Barbara Griggs quotes the French herbalist Maurice Messegué who 'recalls being put in a bath of Lime Flowers and Leaves as a child when he couldn't sleep — with magical results . . .'*

Going to bed

After your bath, if you have a partner who is willing to gently massage your neck and shoulders or feet, do encourage this. If you're on your own, gently massage the bits you can reach, or do some gentle stretching and yawning before you get into bed.

Go to bed in cotton night-wear rather than artificial fibre. Some people find it helpful to put a few drops of an essential oil on your pillow — lavender is particularly good. But don't put the drops where your face will come into direct contact with them; un-diluted essential oils are quite powerful and can cause skin reactions.

*Barbara Griggs, *The Home Herbal: A Handbook of Simple Remedies*, (Jill Norman and Hobhouse, 1982)

Some people find it helpful just before or just after getting into bed to review the day, and then say a firm goodbye to it. Try it: note particularly the things you have enjoyed, however small, and say thank you for them.

Once in bed, relax and let go. Allow your body to be as comfortable as possible, and know that your mind will soon be taking you into sleep. Don't *try* to get to sleep; rather, think of sleep as a friend for whom you have made all the right preparations, and who will arrive in his own good time. Remember that the normal person takes 15-20 minutes to get to sleep, so there's no rush. Only a few happy souls hit sleep when their heads hit the pillow.

If you are still awake after 20 minutes, you have a choice. The stimulus control programme recommends that you get up and *do* something, in a different room. Have a hot drink, or read, or write a letter, until you feel sleepy enough to return to bed. The same rule applies if you wake up in the middle of the night.

If not, the alternative is to stay in bed, but allowing yourself to think of pleasant things. Don't lie there worrying or brooding.

Whichever system you opt for, commit yourself to it for at least three weeks.

Night thoughts

If you body is relaxed but your mind still active, either before going to sleep or after waking up in the small hours, you can train yourself not to focus on anxiety and worry by concentrating on something else.

One method is to play mental games which will keep your mind occupied and possibly rather bored until you drop off. These include things like counting backwards from 100-1, or listing in alphabetical order the names of your friends, or countries, or flowers. You could consider learning a verse or two of a poem before turning in and reciting it to yourself in bed. Or just pick a harmonious line of poetry, and mentally repeat it to yourself over and over.

Listening to the radio has been the resort of many insomniacs, as you will probably have discovered for yourself, but it has the disadvantage that if there's a really interesting programme, you may stay awake to hear it to the end.

If worrying thoughts come into your head, let them go, with the knowledge that you will deal with them at the proper time. As you breathe in, think of peace, tranquillity, calmness entering your system; breathe the worry away.

Another way of dealing with negative or anxious thoughts is not to fight them, but to listen to them in a detached manner as if they were a rather boring radio programme, without trying to find solutions to them.

Mind-games can include images that help to activate the alpha waves that precede sleep: you could take yourself on an imaginary or remembered walk in the country or by the sea. Or take yourself through a film you have really enjoyed.

The more pleasant your thoughts, the more likely you are to relax and get off to sleep. Remember the image of your mind energy: negative thoughts press down on you, while happy ones lift depression away from you. So do thoughts that are not focused on yourself.

I discovered accidentally one wakeful night that praying for other people sent me off in no time. Obviously, the purpose of prayer is not to send you to sleep, nor do I assume that everyone believes in prayer. But if you find your mind returning to your own problems, it may help you to switch your attention to a friend or friends who would benefit from a healing thought from you. If they are ill, don't focus on their illness, but visualize them well and happy, or imagine a stream of healing white or gold light going from your heart to surround them. If you don't visualize clearly, this is not important: simply send them well-wishing thoughts.

If someone pops into your mind who has hurt, insulted, irritated or angered you, send them a healing thought too — they probably need it.

And if you're one of those people who lies awake worrying about the environment, try sending healing thoughts to the planet, to animals, trees and nature, which will do both you and the environment much more good than if you lie there worrying about it.

PART 4

Natural therapies

CHAPTER 1

How natural therapies can help

There is an ever-increasing variety of natural therapies available today, some complementary to orthodox medicine and some alternative; those most appropriate to sleeplessness are described in the next chapter. What they have in common is the principle that we all have our own powers of self-healing. They aim to remove blockages to health and self-healing by restoring harmony and balance, rather than zapping symptoms with drugs which can actually deplete the patient's life force. While their methods vary, they work on the basis that body, mind and emotions are a single, interdependent unit, and that for a healthy system, all three need to be attended to.

As well as curing or relieving medical problems, natural therapies can help you to relax, and can relieve pain and anxiety. Many practitioners are also good counsellors who will provide emotional support to deal with the causes of your insomnia, or with withdrawal from tranquillizers or sleeping pills.

By contrast with conventional medicine, practitioners of natural medicines treat the person rather than the disease, which can involve a multiplicity of approaches, even within the same disciplines. They take into account the patient's personality and lifestyle, recognizing that people vary in their responses to the same treatment. (To be fair to doctors, an increasing number nowadays also aim to treat patients in this holistic way.)

Another difference with conventional medicine is the speed at which treatments work. We have become used to a course of antibiotics, for instance, taking effect very speedily (and there are certainly emergency occasions when antibiotics are very useful). But antibiotics work by suppressing symptoms; natural medicines treat the mind and body which have become sufficiently depleted for bacteria or viruses to flourish, and symptoms are regarded as the body's efforts to defend itself.

This means that restoring health to the whole person can take time. In addition, cure often involves what's known as a healing crisis, when symptoms temporarily worsen as the body starts fighting back. So don't be disappointed if results aren't instant; give whatever therapy you choose at least a couple of months to see how it's affecting you. A good practitioner will be happy to discuss your progress with you after the first few visits, and may then be able to give you an idea of how long treatment will take.

As far as insomnia is concerned, however, since natural treatments can be very relaxing, this is often one of the first symptoms to go.

Choosing a therapy

The plethora of possible therapies can be quite confusing to the new patient. In addition, most individual therapies are taught at a number of different training schools, which often vary in their emphasis and approach. What is important is to find both a therapy and a practitioner that suit you personally. Often the qualities of the practitioner as a person are at least as important as the techniques he or she uses.

The therapies described in the following pages can all be helpful for emotional stress, physical tension and pain, as well as insomnia. If touch is lacking in your life, you might receive particular benefit from a hands-on treatment like osteopathy, chiropractic, aromatherapy, or massage. If you feel taking medication is important or necessary, try homoeopathy or medical herbalism.

Before embarking on a course of treatment it's worth checking out what the practitioner has to offer in addition to any specialization. Some train in more than one discipline, and can advise you on diet or nutritional supplements, or combine treatments like osteopathy and acupuncture.

You may find your practitioner using unusual means of diagnosis: some are trained in iridology, diagnosis through the iris of the eye, which reflects the state of the body: variations in the colour, dark or light spots and so on can indicate organic or functional weaknesses and nutritional deficiencies. Some use kinesiology techniques (see page 150) to test imbalances and nutritional needs; some use dowsing with a pendulum. Some are highly intuitive and can tell a lot about a patient simply by looking at them or touching them.

Assuming your GP is open minded, it's as well to let him or her know that you are seeking additional treatment. Doctors today are conscious of the possible side-effects of tranquillizers and sleeping pills; they don't want patients to become addicted, and many of them recognize the value of alternative forms of reducing anxiety.

However, if you are already taking medication you should discuss this with both your doctor and the natural practitioner you have chosen. Some forms of natural medicine really are alternative rather than complementary to conventional medicine; some herbal medicines, for example, may not be compatible with medical drugs, and the effect of some homoeopathic remedies can be counteracted by drugs like steroids. So you should talk to your doctor before making any changes in or adding to what he or she has already prescribed.

Counselling

Your relationship with and trust in the practitioner can be a major factor in recovery, particularly with a problem like insomnia which so often has an emotional basis. Most alternative practitioners recognize the part played in health by the mind and the emotions; however, this does not mean that every practitioner is necessarily equipped to deal with psychological problems. So you will find some osteopaths, for example, who work purely on physical symptoms; others who encourage patients to discuss their anxieties; and yet others who recognize the emotional factor, but prefer to refer patients to professional counsellors.

For the insomniac the ideal is to find someone who can combine effective physical treatment with a listening ear and emotional understanding. When difficult emotions are not appropriately expressed, the stress around them can become locked into the body; according to one theory when a traumatic event, such as an accident or child abuse, is accompanied by fear, the memory of the event can be 'fixed' in the body by adrenalin. Natural therapies can release these traumatic memories, and sometimes patients find themselves experiencing long-suppressed feelings such as grief, fear, or anger. On such occasions a practitioner who is also a good counsellor can help you to come to terms with and finally free yourself of these past stresses.

Not everyone experiences this kind of dramatic relief, nor is formal counselling always necessary. The touch and caring attention of a massage therapist, osteopath, or healer may gently release the stress built up in the body-mind without the need for deep emotional probing or catharsis. All this will depend on both the therapist's gifts and the patient's own needs and personality.

I have occasionally heard of newly-qualified practitioners who decide to try their hands at 'counselling' and tell patients for instance that they should leave their spouses or their jobs. This is *not* counselling, which is a means of helping patients to clarify issues so that they can make their own decisions. If you want counselling, discuss this with the practitioner first, and find out what experience and training he or she has.

An advantage of good practitioner-counsellors is that they encourage patients to work with them in the healing process, rather than being passive recipients of treatment. As aromatherapist Tricia Donà-Hooker says, 'The most important thing for me is to help the patient exit from being a victim and come into being in control.'

Finding a practitioner

Your choice of practitioner will also, of course, be governed by who is available in your area. The most usual way to find a good one is by personal recommendation; these days some GPs have contacts with reliable non-medical practitioners whom they happily recommend to patients, so it's worth asking your doctor as well as your friends.

Another way is to go to a holistic or natural health clinic, where a number of different therapies are available. A well-run clinic will ensure a high standard of practice, and there should be someone available to interview you and guide you towards the most appropriate therapy. Some clinics are directed by or in collaboration with qualified doctors who can contribute medical advice if necessary. Going to a clinic also has the advantage that if your osteopath, for instance, suspects you have a nutritional or emotional problem, you can be referred to a nutritionist, naturopath, herbalist or counsellor under the same roof.

Some practitioners advertise in the Yellow Pages of the telephone directory, or in local newspapers. Not all professional bodies allow their members to advertise; if you pick a therapist from an advertisement, make sure they are properly qualified and belong to a professional register.

The field of complementary medicine in Britain is at present governed by Common Law, which means that anyone can practise any therapy with very little training and no qualifications. All this is likely to change in 1992 in keeping with European Community regulations, and in preparation for this the natural health professions are tightening up their qualifications and regulations. In the meantime, while some non-registered practitioners are excellent, a few less ethical people have joined the bandwagon.

The addresses of organizations from whom you can obtain lists of qualified practitioners, together with the initials they are entitled to use, are included at the end of each section in the following chapter. All will prefer you to enclose a stamped addressed envelope, and some charge around £1-£2 for directories of their members.

The Institute for Complementary Medicine also keeps registers of practitioners in a variety of fields, and can give you the names of those in your area. The Institute is at 21 Portland Place, London W1N 3AF, tel. 071 636 9543.

Costs

In 1990 a fairly typical first consultation fee for most of the therapies described below was between £20-£25, with £15-£20 for follow-up sessions. Charges are usually lower outside London, where overheads are heavier. Some practitioners charge much higher fees; some make an additional charge for medicines, while aromatherapists have to cover the costs of expensive essential oils.

We have to remember that while medical treatment within the Health Service is 'free', we actually pay for it through our taxes; and if charges seem high, compare the average six-minute consultation provided by an NHS GP with the 30-60 minutes of time and attention a natural practitioner may spend on you. Many operate a sliding scale, so that the fees of better-off patients subsidize pensioners and the less well-off. They don't always advertise the fact; some tell me that when they do, it is the obviously well-to-do who ask for reductions, while pensioners and the less well off pay up willingly.

If money is a problem, it's worth asking whether you can come to some arrangement to make treatment feasible. Some clinics and practitioners offer special days or times for low-income clients, or give concessionary rates to senior citizens and the unemployed. And a smattering of practitioners can be paid through private medical insurance schemes.

CHAPTER 2

The therapies

1. Acupuncture

Acupuncture can be an effective treatment for insomnia, by restoring balance and harmony to the patient's energy system. Return to normal sleep may take several sessions, but some people feel extremely relaxed immediately after or even during a treatment. It can relieve emotional as well as physical pain, calming anxiety and lifting depression. Regarded by most doctors with scepticism only 20 years ago, it is the most widely used complementary therapy within the medical profession, practised by a number of GPs, and increasingly in hospital pain relief clinics.

This ancient Chinese technique is based on the theory that health depends on a harmonious flow of energy, or life force, called *qi* (pronounced *chee*). Qi flows through the body via energy channels called meridians; the twelve main meridians are connected with and named after a physical organ — the heart, lungs, liver, kidneys, and so on — each of which can be affected by a specific emotion. For example, fear affects the kidneys and anger the liver, together with their relevant meridians. Insomnia is usually found to relate to a disruption in the energy flow of the heart meridian, which can be caused by shock, or even by excessive joy.

Too much or too little energy in one or more meridians can give rise to both mental and physical symptoms. Diagnosis therefore focuses on the individual's state of energy rather than specific diseases. Traditional methods include taking a full history, observing the patient's skin colour and possibly tongue, and noting which parts of the body are extra hot or cold. The strength of the meridians is checked through twelve pulses found in the wrists. Over- or under-activity in a meridian can be caused by dietary, physical or emotional factors — often a combination of these — and the acupuncturist's aim is to restore health by restoring the balance. Progress is usually slow and steady, but treatment can sometimes have dramatic effects in releasing traumatic memories, and a few acupuncturists combine their treatment with psychotherapy.

Along the meridians lie hundreds of acupuncture points, tiny gateways into the energy flow, whose Chinese names often indicate their function. Treatment consists of stimulating or sedating the meridians to restore the energy balance, by inserting very fine steel needles into the appropriate points. Whether this is painful or not depends both on the practitioner's touch and the patient's sensitivity. Points that need treatment are usually tender to the touch, and may be slightly painful when the needle is first inserted; as the balance is restored, the pain lessens. Usually only a few points are treated in any one session. The needles may be left in place for 10 to 20 minutes, and the acupuncturist may twiddle them from time to time.

Some people are worried about the possibility of cross-infection through needles. Acupuncturists belonging to the professional associations included in the Council for Acupuncture are bound by a Code of Practice which demands stringent standards of hygiene and sterilization approved by the DHSS; these days many use disposable needles. Some treat the acupuncture points with burning herbs rather than needles, and children may be treated painlessly by stimulating the points with tiny hammers. Acupuncturists all have their favourite methods; some also practise Chinese herbalism in which there is an increasing interest these days.

For insomnia, the acupuncturist may well treat points on the heart meridian, including *Shenmen* ('gate of the spirit'), an important point on the wrist, which is also often used for depression. In traditional Chinese terms the heart is said to be the seat of the mind or spirit, and sleeplessness is caused by the spirit 'rampaging'. In more orthodox terms, treating the heart meridian takes the pressure off the nerves to the heart, which may be over-stimulated.

Acupuncture can be extremely useful in reducing withdrawal

symptoms from tranquillizers, sleeping pills and other drugs including nicotine. Research on heroin addicts in Hong Kong has shown that treatment increases the brain's output of endorphins, reducing pain and lifting the mood. It also stimulates the excretion of drugs from the system. Some acupuncturists prefer patients to come off their pills before starting treatment, since the drugs may counteract the effects of acupuncture.

Finding a practitioner

Directories of qualified acupuncturists can be obtained from:

The British Academy of Western Acupuncture,
Carrick,
Tatchill,
Ellesmere,
Shropshire SY12 9AP
(For doctors, nurses and physiotherapists with five years' clinical practice.)

The British Acupuncture Association,
34 Alderney Street,
London SW1V 4EU
Tel. 071 834 3353/1012
(The first regulatory body for lay and medical acupuncturists, its members have the letters MBAcA or FBAcA after their names.)

The British Medical Acupuncture Society,
The Administrative Officer,
Newton House,
Newton Lane,
Whitley,
Warring WA4 4JA
Tel. 092 573 727
(Medical doctors only.)

The International Register of Oriental Medicine,
Green Hedges House,
Green Hedges Avenue,
East Grinstead,
Sussex RH19 1DZ
Tel. 0342 313106
(Members are graduates of the International College of Oriental Medicine and use the letters MIROM.)

The Register of Traditional Chinese Medicine,
19 Trinity Road,
London N2 8JJ
Tel. 081 883 8431
(An independent register not affiliated to any college, it includes members who have trained in the Far East. Members use the letters MRTCM.)

The Traditional Acupuncture Society,
1 The Ridgeway,
Stratford upon Avon,
Warwickshire CV37 9JL
(Members are graduates of the College of Traditional Chinese Acupuncture (UK) and use the letters MTAcS.)

The Council for Acupuncture,
Panther House,
38 Mount Pleasant,
London WC1X 0AP
Tel. 071 837 8026
(Provides a combined directory of the last four organizations listed above, for a small charge.)

Self-help

Personal contact and a good relationship with the therapist are essential to the success of any natural treatment. However, there are some devices on the market which, though they should not be regarded as substitutes for proper treatment, enable people to treat symptoms at home. They include the AcuHealth, a machine devised by an Australian doctor and acupuncturist, which uses light, painless electric currents instead of needles; it comes with a comprehensive guide to finding and treating the relevant points for a wide range of conditions, including insomnia, restless legs, tension and so on. It costs around £138.00. Details from AcuHealth, 32 Maple Street, London WC2. See also Shiatsu (p. 168).

Further reading

Peter Firebrace, BAcMIROM, and Sandra Hill BAcMIROM, *A Guide to Acupuncture*, (Hamlyn, 1988)

An Introduction to Acupuncture: Handbook of the British Acupuncture Association, (published by the BAA, address above.)

Dr Ruth Lever, *Acupuncture for Everyone*, (Penguin Health, 1987)

Dr Paul Marcus, *Acupuncture: A Patient's Guide*, (Thorsons, 1984)

2. The Alexander Technique

The Alexander Technique can help you sleep better by creating greater physical and mental harmony, enabling you to go through life with less strain. It is a way of learning how to use your body as it was meant to be used — easily, effortlessly, and without tension.

The Technique was developed over eighty years ago by an Australian actor, Frederick Matthias Alexander. Specializing in one-man shows, he was plagued by recurring hoarseness and breathing problems which prevented him from performing. When medical specialists could find nothing wrong with his throat, Alexander decided that there must be something wrong with the way he was using it. He studied himself with the help of mirrors and realized that his voice was being affected by the way he held his head and neck, which in turn related to the tensions in his body.

Over the years he taught himself new habits, not only solving his voice problem but discovering a new mental power and energy. He began teaching his technique to private individuals, including actors; today it is taught at five training schools in Britain, and is very popular among performers of all kinds, who are probably more aware of their bodies than the rest of us.

Small children know instinctively how to hold themselves

correctly, but are soon thrown out of balance from schooldays onwards by things like badly designed school desks and too much sedentary work, as well as the stresses of modern living. Emotions are also reflected in the body; rounded shoulders can develop as a fear response to an over-critical or bullying parent, while over-anxiety can produce a head that thrusts forward instead of balancing easily on top of the spine. These muscular postures tend to become fixed, perpetuating the attitudes of mind they reflect.

Lessons usually last 30 to 45 minutes, during which the teacher helps you gradually to adjust the way you stand, sit and walk, using his or her hands to show the body how it should be, and gently guiding your muscles into new habits. It takes time for habits to be changed, and initially you may need to see a teacher two or three times a week; this is gradually tailed off, so that in time you will only need a lesson every month or two. During this re-education process, tensions are released, the stance becomes more natural, the ribs open up so that you breathe more naturally and deeply, and very often back and neck problems are relieved. As the client becomes more self-aware, he or she is able to go through daily life with less stress.

Despite the gentleness of the technique it can bring about profound changes not only in the body but in the mind, partly through the letting-go of old tensions, and partly through its focus on the present moment. This can result in a new, freer way of responding to stress, anxiety, decision-making and so on. For insomniacs, learning to adopt a different, more flowing attitude to daily activities can be extremely beneficial.

Finding a teacher

For a list of qualified teachers, send s.a.e. to:
The Society of Teachers of the Alexander Technique,
10 London House,
266 Fulham Road,
London SW10 9EL
Tel. 071 351 0828

Further reading

Dr Wilfred Barlow, *The Alexander Principle*, (Arrow Books, 1981)
Michael Gelb, *Body Learning*, (Aurum Press, 1981)

3. Aromatherapy

Aromatherapy must be one of the most delicious ways of treating insomnia. It consists of massage using essential plant oils in a vegetable oil base, and is a wonderful way to experience deep relaxation, excellent for tension and stress-related conditions.

It is more than a pleasant experience, however. The essential oils are distilled from the flowers, leaves or roots of plants with specific curative properties. Their volatine elements are absorbed through the skin into the bloodstream, and into both the body and brain through the membranes at the back of the nose. They can affect the organs and glands within the body, and have a direct effect on mood, since they reach the parts of the brain controlling the emotions. So there are oils that can simultaneously calm you, clear your brain, and lift depression, as well as healing your physical body.

In France aromatherapy constitutes a complete system of alternative medicine; in the UK it has until recently been more associated with beauty care, since the oils are often used as an adjunct to a general massage or facial. However, practised by a qualified aromatherapist, there are medical conditions like rheumatic pains that it can certainly ease. Robert Tisserand, Britain's leading aromatherapist, points out that the combination of massage, essential oils and relaxation can boost the immune system; his book *Aromatherapy for Everyone* (Penguin Books, 1988) includes a variety of case histories illustrating its various therapeutic uses.

These days aromatherapy is used in some hospitals and hospices, largely at the instigation of nurses, who recognize the value of healing touch. Within the medical context it does not replace drugs, but it does enhance their effects so that smaller doses can be prescribed.[*]

[*]Helen Passant, 'A Holistic Approach in the Ward', *Nursing Times* (24-30 January 1990)

A qualified aromatherapist will first take clients through a questionnaire to check on their medical history and specific needs, looking in the case of insomnia for its emotional and physical causes before choosing what combination of oils to use. One of the beauties of aromatherapy is that each oil has several properties, so that you can be treated on several levels at once.

The treatment itself can take up to an hour, sometimes longer, and usually the whole body will be massaged. Some people find themselves going to sleep on the massage table; some find that in this relaxed state they can talk out their problems with the therapist. And because scents can trigger the emotions and the memory, clients may find themselves experiencing an emotional release during or after a treatment. 'You release the tensions, and also bring out things that people may have buried,' says aromatherapist Tricia Donà-Hooker. 'When people allow things to come up in them, they can be recognized and dealt with.'

Aromatherapists may well be able to help you come off sleeping pills or tranquillizers, using oils that can both calm you and cleanse your system of the drugs; like other natural thera-pists they will want you to get your doctor's agreement first.

The choice of oils will depend on the individual's physical and mental state. In *Aromatherapy for Everyone* Robert Tisserand describes how he helped an elderly widow suffering from depression and nightmares, one of whose children had died from a heroin overdose. Aromatherapy massage using a blend of frankincense, bergamot, clary sage and jasmine gradually cured her of her nightmares and depression, and enabled her to give up her nightly sleeping pill.

Your aromatherapist may also suggest nutritional changes, or supplements, Bach Flower Remedies or herbal remedies to take at home.

Self-help

A full aromatherapy treatment must be given by a professional, but your therapist may make up a mixture of oils for use at home, perhaps to rub into painful joints or as a relaxant in the bath. Oils can also be inhaled, either by putting a drop or two on a handkerchief, or as an inhalation in boiling water.

You can buy essential oils in health food shops and pharmacies, and from herbalists; make sure they are reputable brands. Good quality oils include those made by Body Treats, Fleur, Neal's Yard Apothecary, Shirley Price and Robert Tisserand. Some shops make up their own cheaper brands which may be of inferior quality or heavily diluted; they smell nice but don't do much for you. Unfortunately, good oils can be expensive; prices vary according to the rarity of the plant. Blue Camomile, for instance, which is excellent for insomnia, costs around £40 for a small bottle.

More moderately priced oils which are helpful for insomnia are firstly lavender, which is extremely versatile; it's good for burns, insect bites, period problems and strengthening the immune system, among other properties. Neroli, marjoram, lemongrass, and linden (lime) blossom are all soothing; geranium helps to create balance and harmony; melissa oil is uplifting, and ylang-ylang will help lift depression. (Ylang-ylang also has a reputation as an aphrodisiac, so using it for a bedtime massage might not lead immediately to sleep.) Any of these oils can be used in the bath. To aid sleep, you can also put two or three drops on your pillow or on a handkerchief to sniff if you wake in the night.

If you have a partner or friend who will give your neck, shoulders and spine a gentle massage, you can make up your own massage oil. Use three or four drops of a single aroma-therapy oil or two drops each of two oils in an egg-cup full of a base oil such as sweet almond or grape-seed.

If you make up larger amounts remember that once mixed, they will not retain their properties for very long. Keep the mixture in a dark, air-tight bottle and use it within three months. Don't use the same oil or oil mixture consecutively for too long, as it may lose its initial impact.

Caution: Essential oils are extremely potent, and should not be used neat on your skin; you could have an allergic reaction or, like the man who unwittingly used neat rosemary oil on his head for baldness, you could suffer from even more severe insomnia and 'mental chatter'.

Never take aromatherapy oils internally (unless prescribed by a medical aromatherapist.

Finding an aromatherapist

Registers of qualified practitioners are available from:

The Association of Tisserand Aromatherapists (ATA),
PO Box 746,
Brighton BN1 3BN

The International Federation of Aromatherapists,
4 Eastmearn Road,
W. Dulwich, London SE21 8HA

Further reading

Patricia Davis, *Aromatherapy, An A-Z*, (C.W. Daniel, 1988)
Shirley Price, *Practical Aromatherapy*, (Thorsons, 1987)
Maggie Tisserand, *Aromatherapy for Women*, (Thorsons 1985)
Robert Tisserand, *The Art of Aromatherapy*, (C.W. Daniel, 1977)
Robert Tisserand, *Aromatherapy for Everyone*, (Penguin Books, 1988)

4. Bach Flower Remedies

Bach Flower Remedies were the discovery of Dr Edward Bach (pronounced 'Batch', though a lot of people understandably pronounce it as they do the composer's name). A physician of Welsh descent, highly intuitive and sensitive, he spent his working life seeking ever purer methods of healing. After qualifying at University College Hospital he worked as a pathologist and bacteriologist, and then took up homoeopathy.

He came to the conclusion that illnesses are caused by negative mental states which, if prolonged, damage physical health. Conversely happiness, based on being in touch with one's higher self and life's purpose, allows the body to return to its natural state of good health.

In 1934 Dr Bach left his Harley Street practice to seek in the countryside plants that were appropriate to specific mental states. By holding his hand over plants to sense their energy, he intuitively discovered 38 remedies for different states of mind, testing them on himself and others.

He listed seven main moods: fear, uncertainty, lack of interest in the present, loneliness, over-sensitivity to influences, despair, and over-concern for others. He subdivided these, for example finding seven remedies for different kinds of fear including mimulus for fear of known causes, and aspen for fear of the unknown. He also created a thirty-ninth, Rescue Remedy, composed of five remedies, to be used for physical and mental shock, accidents and traumas.

Today his work continues at the small house in Oxfordshire where he finally settled. Here the remedies are still prepared according to the method he discovered one day while walking through a dew-sprinkled field. Summer flowers and tree blossoms are picked at their best and the heads are floated in a bowl of spring water in full sunlight. After three hours the water starts to bubble and sparkle, 'impregnated with the vital energy of the flowers'.

The fluid is then strained and poured into a bottle with a small amount of brandy as a preservative. This, known as the stock, reaches the public in small brown bottles with dropper tops. To take them they are then further diluted, two drops to a small bottle of water. People are usually recommended to take from this four drops, four times a day.

There is no known scientific reason why these remedies should work, but the quantity of grateful letters received at the Bach Centre attests to the fact that they do. Without ever having advertised, the Centre is constantly busy, making and distributing the remedies, giving personal consultations and answering enquiries from all over the world.

Bach Remedies can be effective by themselves, and are an excellent adjunct to any other treatment you may be having. They can be made up in combinations of up to six remedies, since people often suffer from more than one symptom: some practitioners find it more effective to prescribe one at a time. Results can be instant or may take a few months; they occur so naturally that people sometimes only notice the change in themselves much later, looking back.

With their healing effect on mental states, the remedies can be very helpful with insomnia. Since they are chosen according to the personality, symptoms and attitudes of the sufferer, different remedies will suit different people. For example, for insomnia caused by a sudden bereavement, suitable remedies might include star of Bethlehem for shock, honeysuckle for a tendency to live in the past and perhaps chicory for self-pity. Willow is good for resentment, and holly for anger, olive for exhaustion of mind and body. A workaholic secretary who suffered from migraines as well as insomnia was prescribed oak for over-conscientiousness and olive for her exhaustion; after taking them for two months her migraines and insomnia had totally cleared up.

Bach Remedies can also help people coming off tranquillizers and sleeping pills by dealing with any old anxieties and worries that re-emerge during withdrawal.

The remedies are very effective with babies and children, and are totally harmless; if the 'wrong' remedy is taken it will simply have no effect. Obviously, a child who is suffering should have a physical check-up, but where there is no obvious medical condition Bach Remedies may supply a gentle and effective solution. One little boy of 20 months had been 'cranky, nervous and not sleeping' ever since falling from his cot two months earlier. His mother took him to her doctor, who used natural as well as orthodox treatments. After finding no physical damage, the doctor prescribed star of Bethlehem for the shock of the fall. Only two days later, the child was his normal happy self.

Not too many doctors would take the remedies seriously, but some natural practitioners use them in conjunction with their own treatment, and can choose remedies for you on the basis of your symptoms or by dowsing with a pendulum. The Dr Edward Bach Centre sees people by appointment, and will make up remedies. No charge is made for a personal or postal consultation.

Self-help

Anyone can treat themselves, with the help of Dr Bach's booklet *The Twelve Healers and Other Remedies* (available from the Bach Centre); however, it can be hard to see oneself clearly enough to decide which remedies to take and initially it is best to get advice from an expert. As you become familiar with the remedies, it becomes easier to self-prescribe, and also to recommend them for your friends and family.

Bach Flower Remedies can be bought at many health food shops and pharmacies and some homoeopathic pharmacies at around £1.80 for a stock bottle, or slightly more cheaply direct from the Dr Edward Bach Centre, Mount Vernon, Sotwell, Wallingford, Oxon OX10 0PZ, tel. 0491 39489; they will also supply literature on using the remedies.

Further reading

Dr Edward Bach, *The Twelve Healers and Other Remedies*, (C.W. Daniel, 1989). (How to choose and use the remedies)

Philip M. Chancellor, *Handbook of the Bach Flower Remedies*, (C.W. Daniel, 1971). (Contains numerous case histories relating to each remedy)

Mechthild Scheffer, *Bach Flower Therapy*, (Thorsons, 1986)

5. Homoeopathy

Homoeopathy is another complete system of medicine which can treat insomniacs on many levels, including the body, mind, and energy system. Developed during the eighteenth century by a German doctor, Samuel Hahnemann, it is based on giving minute doses of natural substances (plants, bee stings and so on) which, instead of suppressing symptoms, encourage the body to fight back.

The choice of remedies is based on the supposition that 'like cures like': if you give certain substances, for example quinine, to a healthy person, that person will develop the symptoms of a fever; therefore giving it to someone feverish will produce a cure. (Thus one of many possible remedies for insomnia is caffeine.)

Over 20 years Hahnemann built up a complete repertoire of symptoms brought on by different remedies. He also experimented with making finer and finer dilutions of these remedies; at each stage of the dilution he subjected the solution to 'succussion'; banging it repeatedly on a hard surface to ensure the drops were thoroughly mixed. Without succussion, the remedies were ineffective, and it has continued to be an essential part of the process of making up homoeopathic medicines. Continuing with dilution and succussion, Hahnemann ended up with a finished product of so high a potency that no molecules remained of the original substance.

It is this last fact that has made many scientists and medical doctors highly sceptical about homoeopathy, although its effectiveness has been shown time and again, both in individual patients and in some scientifically conducted trials. The reason why these highly diluted potencies work probably lies in the field of energy medicine, which is a very new area of exploration.

Whatever the scientific explanation, a number of medically trained doctors these days take further training in homoeopathy, which they find gentler and safer than many conventional drugs, and there are a few homoeopathic hospitals where you can be treated under the NHS. There are also numbers of non-medical homoeopaths who, while they have not gone through medical school, have usually taken a longer training in homoeopathy itself than qualified doctors. There used to be considerable friction between medical and non-medical practitioners, but these days the two groups are beginning to draw closer.

At the first consultation, the practitioner will ask the patient all kinds of questions: about his or her emotions, tastes in food, dreams, feelings and attitudes, and so on, as well as about any physical symptoms. The remedy or remedies will only be prescribed when a complete picture of the person has been built up.

The homoeopathic treatment of insomnia, says a homoeopath, 'is not something you can treat in isolation. You really do have to look at the whole person.' Since insomnia is often part of a whole conglomerate of symptoms, often going back to patterns developed in childhood or adolescence, or resulting from some later trauma, remedies will be chosen to deal both with the symptoms and their underlying causes.

For people coming off sleeping pills or other addictions homoeopathic remedies help to strengthen the system at the same time as clearing it. If during withdrawal people find themselves re-experiencing the emotional problems that caused them to become addicted in the first place, a good homoeopath will also supply reassurance and counselling, or refer patients for counselling if necessary.

Homoeopathy is excellent and safe for children and babies,

who respond to it very well. Since the remedies take effect over time, there are some risks in trying to treat yourself long-term, but a child who swallows a bottle of homoeopathic tablets in one go will come to no harm.

Self-help

Although there are some homoeopathic sleeping pills on the market, they may not be suitable for everyone. The *Materia Medica*, the homoeopath's 'bible', includes many pages describing a vast range of types of insomnia ('racing thoughts', 'early waking', 'fear', 'anxiety', 'worse in morning' and so on) and specific remedies for each. So it isn't possible to recommend a blanket remedy for everyone. A homoeopatic pharmacist may be willing to make up a remedy for you, but would probably advise you to consult a professional homoeopath as well.

However, if you are interested in using homoeopathy for first aid at home, for yourself or your children (and pets), there are some good books around, including *Everybody's Guide to Homoeopathic Medicines* and *The Family Guide to Homoeopathy* (details below). Look out, too, for weekend or evening courses on homoeopathy, likely to be advertised at your local health shop.

Finding a homoeopath

Registers can be obtained from the following organizations:

The British Homoeopathic Association,
27a Devonshire Street,
London W1N 1RJ
Tel. 071 935 2163
(Has a list of doctors who have qualified at the Faculty of Homoeopathy, with MFHom or FFHom after their names.)

The Society of Homoeopaths,
2 Artizan Road,
Northampton NN1 4HU
Tel. 0604 21400
(Will provide a list of registered homoeopaths who have trained at various approved colleges, and who use the initials RSHom.)

Further reading

Dr Anne Clover, *Homoeopathy: A Patient's Guide*, (Thorsons, 1984)

Stephen Cummings & Dana Ullman, *Everybody's Guide to Homoeopathic Medicines*, (Gollancz, 1989)

Drs Sheila & Robin Gibson, *Homoeopathy for Everyone*, (Penguin Health, 1987)

Dr Andrew Lockie, *The Family Guide to Homeopathy: The Safe Form of Medicine for the Future*, (Elm Tree Books, 1989)

Sarah Richardson, RSHom, *A Guide to Homeopathy*, (Hamlyn, 1988)

Dana Ullman, *Homoeopathy: Medicine for the 21st Century*, (Thorsons, 1989)

6. Kinesiology

Kinesiology is a way of examining and rebalancing the whole person. It can help the insomniac by identifying and correcting imbalances in body and mind, using a series of muscle tests and other techniques. It was the brainchild of an American chiropractor, Dr George Goodheart, who found that by testing the strength of specific muscles in a systematic way, it is possible to evaluate the patient's state as a whole: nutritional/chemical, emotional, musculo-skeletal and energetic.

This system, which Dr Goodheart called Applied Kinesiology, is taught in the UK as Systematic Kinesiology; some practitioners refer to themselves as systematic kinesiologists, some as kinesiologists and some as kinesiotherapists. There are also simplified forms such as Touch for Health and Balanced Health, which are intended only for family use or as an adjunct to another therapy.

Some practitioners work purely as kinesiologists, while a number use kinesiology combined with other skills. An extremely basic form consists of testing whether a person's arm becomes weaker or stronger in reaction to certain foods, substances, or thoughts. This can look impressive; it is fascinating to see how an anxious thought, for instance, or a sugar-lump in the mouth, can cause someone's arm instantly to weaken, while a happy thought or a bite of an apple will strengthen it. However, serious kinesiologists regard this as a party trick: properly practised kinesiology is a great deal more complex.

It is based on the knowledge of a whole series of connections between particular muscles, organs, glands and bodily systems, including the acupuncture meridians and the circuitry of the brain and nervous system. So for correct treatment it's important to go to somebody who has done a reasonable amount of training, as well as being a good counsellor.

For insomnia, says kinesiologist Maggie La Tourelle: 'The first consideration would be to look for a balance in life, including nutrition, exercise and fresh air. Is the person in over-load or under-load? Some people don't sleep because they are not doing enough in their lives, and are not satisfied or motivated; if they're not expelling healthy energy during the day this can disturb them at night. Or are they working too hard? I would probably find all this out through counselling. I would look at the various stressors — emotional, work, environmental, chemical and so on, and identify where the stress is, both by counselling and by muscle testing.'

Muscle-testing is a way of asking the body non-verbal questions, to which its reactions give a truthful reply. To detect nutritional deficiencies and allergic reactions, the kinesiologist tests the strength of particular muscles in response to the patient's contact with items of food, vitamin and mineral samples and so on.

What is actually being tested is the brain's response to two things at once: holding the muscle in a particular position, together with another factor, like food. If there is a stress caused by the food, the brain cannot respond to the muscle test, and the muscle weakens. Items you need will strengthen the muscles, while items that are not therapeutic will weaken them. This is very useful if you are uncertain what supplements to take; Dr Goodheart once tested a film star who was taking 56 nutrients, and found she only needed four!

The kinesiologist can also 'ask' the body which of the various aspects — emotional, structural and so on — needs treating first, and whether any other treatment is needed. Once the areas of weakness have been discovered, he or she applies various techniques to strengthen and rebalance the body and its circuits. These include light massage on body reflexes to stimulate the lymphatic and vascular systems, and touching or holding the meridians and acupuncture points to release energy. Treatment includes nutritional and dietary advice; the kinesiologist may also recommend Bach Flower Remedies.

An important aspect of kinesiology consists of techniques for creating balance in the brain, both between the left and right hemispheres, and also the forebrain (to do with future projects) and the back-brain (to do with memory and the past), which are often in conflict with each other. If the insomnia is caused by an over-stress on the logical hemisphere and neglect of the intuitive side, the balance is restored by using a number of brain integration techniques. Brian Butler, director of the Association of Systematic Kinesiologists, suggests drawing a large 'lazy 8' (the figure 8 lying on its side); then keeping your nose pointed towards the centre, follow the 8 round with your eyes for a minute or two. This can improve concentration and memory, among other benefits.

Another helpful technique, Emotional Stress Release, gently clears emotional trauma. By placing his or her hands on the patient's temples, the kinesiologist takes the charge out of an emotionally charged event, so that the memory is no longer disturbing. Clients can be taught to do this for themselves at home, which could be very helpful if a memory keeps you awake at night.

Kinesiologists may suggest other physical or mental exercises to do at home, including writing or repeating affirmations (positive statements), so that the balance can be maintained. 'I think that's very important,' says Maggie La Tourelle. 'So that people know they can leave the therapist's room and do something for themselves.'

Muscle testing can also be used to test for geopathic stress; for this the kinesiologist would need to test you on-site at home.

Finding a kinesiologist

A list of qualified members can be obtained from:

The Association of Systematic Kinesiologists,
39 Browns Road,
Surbiton,
Surrey KT5 8ST
Tel. 081 399 3215

Further reading

Tom and Carole Valentine, *Applied Kinesiology*, (Thorsons, 1985)

7. *Massage*

Massage is another helpful and enjoyable way of dealing with the stresses associated with insomnia, particularly for people who find it difficult to relax. To lie on a couch having your body caringly tended to can ease away all kinds of muscular and mental tensions. Touch and relaxation are healing in themselves; in addition, massage stimulates the circulation of blood and lymph, boosting the flow of oxygen and essential nutrients in the blood and also helping the body to free itself of waste toxins. This can be particularly beneficial for problems like rheumatism and arthritis.

It's interesting how massage has taken off over the last decade in Britain, since the British are not famous for appreciating the power of touch. Some men, in particular, seem to find it hard to understand that touch can be intimate and healing without having to lead to a sexual clinch, and in some areas massage is only slowly losing its erotic associations. Yet it is one of the most ancient and most natural forms of therapy, practised since ancient times in the East, and adopted by Ancient Greek physicians as a valid aspect of medicine. It is now beginning to come into its own in the West, and is regarded as a valid therapy by both natural practitioners and hospital nurses.

Everyone can benefit from massage, from the very young to the very old. Baby massage is becoming quite popular; gently stroking your baby all over is not only soothing but will help him or her to grow up with a good sense of self-acceptance. Old people can benefit greatly from touch, and are often starved of it — a lack that can certainly contribute to insomnia. In addition, massage with a good oil helps to keep their skin strong and supple.

There are various methods of massage; probably the best-known is Swedish Massage which uses a variety of techniques to relieve stress, encourage circulation, take the tension out of tight muscles and break down fat. Becoming popular today is Intuitive Massage, which is less rigidly structured and also takes into account the body's energy system.

A professional massage can take an hour or longer, and is a very pleasant experience. These days massage therapists often use aromatherapy oils in their massage oils.

Self-help

Many people find that giving a massage is a soothing as receiving one; more than one massage therapist has told me that focusing their attention on the other person is like a form of meditation. Couples attending massage courses find that it brings them closer; non-sexual touch can have a loving quality that can feed back into your sex life. And for couples going through a bad patch, emotionally or sexually, learning massage together can sometimes break through barriers that talking can't.

Anyone can give a massage to their child, partner or relative, particularly concentrating on the neck and shoulders; but if you are untrained, keep your touch gentle — particularly if you massage someone's head. It's even nicer if you use a pleasantly scented aromatherapy oil. If you want to take it further, look out for evening classes or weekend courses. You can learn a great deal from the thorough and well-illustrated *Book of Massage* (details below) which gives instructions for intuitive massage, shiatsu and reflexology, with sections on massaging babies and old people, and on the energy system and centres.

Massaging the feet

This can also be extraordinarily soothing, mentally and physically; among other benefits it draws tension away from the head, helping to calm an over-active mind. If you have a partner who is willing to massage your feet, try it after getting into bed; you may well find yourself drifting off to sleep.

Foot massage is also a very good way to get a fractious baby to settle down — just gently stroke the feet for a few minutes after a bath. Of course, with babies, you can do this at any time of day.

Massaging yourself

Self-massage is obviously not as satisfactory as having someone doing it for you, but it can still be quite soothing. Starting with your head, go down whatever bits of you you can reach, gently pressing and releasing with your palms and fingers. Then use your hands to lightly brush yourself down, smoothing out the energy field around you.

Simply massaging your hands and fingers can also release quite a lot of tension. Try it: you may find yourself yawning.

Finding a therapist

At the time of writing there is a large number of massage schools throughout the country, but no central register; the Institute for Complementary Medicine (21, Portland Place, London W1N 3AF) is compiling a register of massage therapists country-wide. There are massage practitioners at most holistic clinics.

If you choose someone through an advertisement, people calling themselves massage therapists or massage practitioners are likely to be genuine.

Further reading

Nigel Dawes and Fiona Harrold, *Massage Cures*, (Thorsons, 1990)
Lucinda Lidell, *The Book of Massage*, (Ebury Press, 1984)

8. Medical herbalism

Herbal medicine has been used by mankind throughout the ages and all over the world, and is growing in popularity today in response to concern about drugs, and the desire for more natural forms of medication. Herbalists, like any other natural practitioners, feel that relying on herbs simply as tranquillizers is much the same as relying on medical drugs unless you also deal with the causes of your insomnia. The herbalist's aim is not merely to treat symptoms, but to prescribe medicines that will improve general vitality, clear the system of toxins, and restore balance and harmony; good sleep then comes about naturally.

Many modern drugs are based on plants: aspirin is extracted from willow, and digitalis from the foxglove, for instance. What modern science has done is to isolate from these plants, the 'active ingredient' that provides relief or cure. What it has overlooked in this process is that each herb contains a *balance* of ingredients which counteract any side effects from the active ingredient taken in isolation. They also contain health-promoting vitamins and trace elements. Herbalism is therefore generally very safe and properly prescribed medicines have no side-effects. It is true, of course, that some herbs are harmful, and you should go to someone who has been properly trained.

Herbalists treat much the same range of problems as GPs, and their diagnostic techniques resemble those of medical doctors, using the same equipment for testing blood pressure and so on. As well as assessing symptoms, practitioners evaluate the overall balance of the body's various systems to ascertain underlying disharmonies, and they prescribe on the basis of the whole person rather than symptoms alone. Therefore, as with homoeopathy and other natural medicines, prescriptions for the same disease will vary for individual patients. Different herbs would be appropriate, for instance, for sleeplessness caused by anxiety, digestive problems, hormonal imbalance, and so on.

For insomnia, the herbalist would want to find out what is contributing to lack of sleep. Practitioners look into the patient's lifestyle, including exercise and nutrition, and will recommend a healthy, wholefood diet; treatment is regarded as a co-operative effort in which patients play their part by making any changes that are indicated.

Medicines are usually dispensed in liquid form as tinctures. Herbal medicine can act quite fast, particularly when patients pay attention to a good diet. In chronic cases, however, it can take time to restore health as the medicines work gently and thoroughly, both detoxifying the patient's system and building up his or her strength.

There is a wide choice of herbs that aid sleep, some of them listed in Part 3, Chapter 4.

Finding a herbalist

A register of qualified medical herbalists is obtainable from:

The National Institute of Medical Herbalism,
41 Hatherley Road,
Winchester,
Hampshire SO22 6RR.

Self-help

Herbal medicines can be useful to try out at home for minor health problems in adults and children, and you can learn to use them from a number of books including those listed below. If you take a herbal remedy for a chronic condition, you can expect some improvement within two or three days, but it may take two or more weeks to get the full effect. So take any remedy for a month to give it a fair trial, and when you do improve, taper off gradually. Herbs are not truly addictive, but since they act upon the central nervous system they should not be taken regularly for weeks on end.

Suppliers of herbs by post include:

Baldwins,
173 Walworth Road,
London SE17 1RW
Tel. 071 703 5550

Gerard House,
3 Wickham Road,
Bournemouth, BH7 6JX
Tel: 0202 434116

D. Napier & Son,
1 Teviot Place,
Edinburgh EH1 1HA
Tel. 031 225 5542

Further reading

Barbara Griggs, *The Home Herbal: A Handbook of Simple*

Remedies, (Jill Norman and Hobhouse, 1982)
Richard Mabey (ed.), *The Complete New Herbal*, (Elm Tree Books, 1988)
Simon Y. Mills MA, ENIMH, *The A-Z of Modern Herbalism*, (Thorsons, 1989)

9. The Metamorphic Technique

The Metamorphic Technique is another highly relaxing treatment which can have you nodding off during a session. In addition, people who have regular sessions find themselves changing for the better, becoming better able to cope with problems and clear about what they want in life. The tensions and anxieties leading to sleeplessness can drop away in the process.

The technique is a very gentle form of massage of the feet, hands and head — principally the feet. It is believed to stimulate the receiver's powers of self-healing by releasing emotional blocks. It was developed by an English naturopath, Robert St John, after studying reflexology. Reflexology works on the whole foot and on physical symptoms; in the reflexology system the inner side of the foot, from the big toe to the heel, represents the head and spine. St John discovered intuitively that this area also represents the period of conception, gestation and birth, and that gently massaging it can release emotional traumas experienced during this vital time.

Children can benefit enormously from the Metamorphic Technique, and often enjoy giving sessions to other people. A good deal of work has been done on children with Down's Syndrome and other problems; the technique can also soothe children who are hyperactive or highly strung. Adult stroke patients, and people with nervous disorders have also benefited from it. The technique is not a form of medicine and its practitioners do not claim cures; it seems to have the effect of allowing the person to reach his or her full potential, whatever that potential happens to be.

Self-help and further information

The Metamorphic Technique is easy to learn and practise, with your friends, partner or children; sessions should not be given more than once a week. It's also possible to treat yourself, though this is never as relaxing as receiving a treatment from someone else.

Instructions are given in *The Metamorphic Technique* by Gaston St Pierre and Debbie Shapiro (Element Books, 1982). Personal tuition is advisable to start with, however; as well as the very simple technique, practitioners need to learn to adopt a detached attitude, unconcerned with getting results — something not everyone finds easy.

The Metamorphic Association runs regular workshops in London, and workshops are also organized in other centres. For details of workshops and a list of practitioners, send an s.a.e. to:

The Metamorphic Association,
67 Ritherdon Road,
London SW17 8QE
Tel. 081 672 5951

10. Natural Reconnective Therapy

Although only recently introduced to Britain, Natural Reconnective Therapy is believed to have its origins in Ancient Egypt. It is a method of using gentle pressure on different points of the body with the main focus on the connective tissue, which feels like a deep and very relaxing massage. Practitioners also use their thumbs to separate and realign the vertebrae, totally painlessly.

Like other natural therapies, it aims to restore the body's self-healing mechanism, and it can treat not only difficult musculo-skeletal problems like whiplash injury and slipped discs, but a variety of other conditions.

Natural Reconnective Therapy can help the sleepless not just by dealing with specific aches and pains but by erasing stress from the body. The treatment involves the unique theory that the body contains a system of memory banks, specific places in the connective tissue where tensions are stored. For example, a nervous system memory bank and a heart memory bank can be found in the shoulder-blade areas. Memory banks can be likened to cassette tapes on which every trauma is recorded; if one becomes full up, physical or emotional ill-health follows. An important part of the treatment therefore consists of a specific method of massaging the appropriate points, wiping out the effects of stress. Thus treating the nervous system memory can erase the effects of emotional trauma and stress which deprive so many people of sleep.

Patients are also recommended to adopt the Way of Life system of eating, which helps to restore the body's natural harmony. (See 'The Timing of Meals', Part 3, Chapter 3.)

Further information

For details send s.a.e. to:

The Natural Reconnective Therapy School,
P.O. Box 630
Hove,
East Sussex BN3 6BQ

11. Naturopathy

Naturopaths not only advise on nutrition but look at their patients' whole lifestyle, including their working life and any anxieties causing particular stress, and will work with patients to deal with the problems underlying insomnia. Many naturopaths are also trained in osteopathy (described in the next section), which helps to relieve structural and muscular tensions and pain.

Sometimes called nature cure, naturopathy is one of the best established forms of natural and holistic medicine; it has had its followers in Britain since well before the Second World War. It is based on the principle that the body has its own restorative powers, and under the right conditions will heal itself. The right conditions for good health include nutrition, exercise, relaxation, a balanced and unstressed musculo-skeletal system, and a positive outlook on life. Treatment therefore consists chiefly of removing impediments to health rather than adding extras, although naturopaths may use some herbal and homoeopathic preparations as well as nutritional supplements when appropriate to individual needs.

Practitioners may advocate fasting, to rid the body of accumulated poisons — either a complete fast, or a few days on fruit or fruit juices. Fasting doesn't suit everyone, and the naturopath will take your personal needs and system into account before recommending it. Hydrotherapy (water cure) is also traditionally associated with naturopathy, including treatments such as encouraging the circulation around arthritic joints by alternate applications of hot and cold water, or using sitz baths to improve the circulation in the abdominal area. More elaborate forms of hydrotherapy are applied at some health farms.

Naturopaths will also advise on appropriate exercise and relaxation techniques, and support you in making changes to your lifestyle.

Finding a naturopath

Literature and registers of qualified practitioners can be obtained from:

The General Council and Register of Naturopaths,
Frazer House,
6 Netherhall Gardens,
London NW3 5RR
Tel. 071 435 8728
(Members have ND (Diploma in Naturopathy) and/or DO, MRN after their names.)

The British Register of Naturopaths,
1 Albemarle Road,
The Mount,
York YO2 1EN
Tel. 0904 23693
(Members do not use initials.)

Further reading

Roger Newman Turner, *Naturopathic Medicine*, (Thorsons, 1984)

12. Osteopathy and Chiropractic

Manipulative techniques can often help insomniacs, and not only by relieving pain in the back or other joints; treatment can be an excellent stress reliever. Insomnia, headaches, migraines and general tension are, for example, often caused or exacerbated by problems in the vertebrae of the neck, which both the osteopath and the chiropractic can relieve or cure.

Both these methods of treating the musculo-skeletal system (the bones, muscles and joints) are becoming increasingly accepted by orthodox medicine. The two therapies were evolved independently in America towards the end of the nineteenth century, and there are variations between them, although some techniques are common to both. There are also variations between the techniques used by practitioners from different training schools.

This is particularly the case with chiropractic: members of the British Chiropractic Association have undergone a full-time four-year course which is medically and academically oriented and now has degree status; many take their own X-rays. Members of the Institute of Pure Chiropractic have trained at the part-time McTimoney School, whose teaching is based on a very gentle but effective technique developed by an Englishman, John McTimoney; as well as training in anatomy and physical techniques, the school encourages the development and use of the intuition.

Both osteopathy and chiropractic are based on the principle that the health of the spine has a profound effect on overall well-being. The spinal cord is an extension of the brain, and connects with all the organs of the body via the circulatory and nervous systems. So although people generally seek these therapies for back and joint pain, they can be beneficial for a wide range of problems as diverse as asthma, migraine, indigestion, hiatus hernia, pre-menstrual tension and so on. Some practitioners are good counsellors; some also take a particular interest in nutrition, and can advise you on diet and supplements, particularly those who have also trained in naturopathy.

Adjusting the vertebrae is not usually painful, and the effects can be extremely relaxing. One woman who had barely slept for four years after injuring her neck in a car accident eventually visited a chiropractor; after treatment she fell asleep for several hours, and subsequently returned to a normal sleep pattern.

Nowadays quite elderly people are turning to these therapies for help with arthritic and back pain with good results. Manipulation may not cure the arthritis, but it can relieve the pressure on arthritic joints and improve the circulation of blood around them, helping to remove toxic waste. Practitioners have a variety of techniques at their disposal, as well as, or instead of, actual manipulation which might be over-traumatic for the old or those in very severe pain. Soft tissue techniques (specific ways of massaging the muscles) also help to realign joints, relax over-tense bodies, and boost the circulation of blood and lymphatic drainage.

A woman in her forties went to an osteopath specifically for her insomnia; for about a year she had been waking at three in the morning, only falling asleep again when it was nearly time to get up. She was not under any special stress, but was overweight and suffered from indigestion. The osteopath first treated her for muscle tension and restriction in the shoulder girdle; in the next two months, as these tensions relaxed, she began to return to normal sleep. The osteopath then went on to treat her back, pelvis and abdomen, relieving her other problems of indigestion and painful periods.*

Cranial osteopathy, or cranio-sacral therapy

This is an extremely gentle approach to manipulation practised by some osteopaths and chiropractors. It is based on the connection between the cranium (the skull) and the sacrum, the shield-shaped bone at the base of the spine.

Practitioners often work simply by placing a hand gently on the relevant parts of the spine, relieving tensions and encouraging the flow of cerebro-spinal fluid, which nourishes the spinal cord. This is extremely relaxing in itself, as well as curative. They may also treat the skull and jaw, often an area of much tension.

Cranial treatment can be very helpful for both babies and mothers after a difficult birth. A cranial check-up after birth might prevent a lot of 'inexplicable' problems in babies.

*Edward Triance, DO, *Osteopathy: A Patient's Guide*, (Thorsons, 1986)

A number of cranial osteopaths are very intuitive, and can tune into the emotional origins of their patients' pain, helping to heal mind and body simultaneously.

Finding a practitioner

Some GPs have a good relationship with manipulative therapists and will refer patients to them. Some doctors practise manipulative techniques themselves. Don't go to anyone without proper qualifications. Details of qualified practitioners can be obtained from:

The British Chiropractic Association,
10 Greycoat Place,
London SW1P 1SB
Tel. 071 222 8866
(For Register of British Chiropractors trained at the Anglo-European College of Chiropractic in Bournemouth, who use the initials DC. In future they will be able to use BSc.)

The Institute of Pure Chiropractic,
PO Box 126,
Oxford OX1 1UF
Tel. 0865 246687
(For register of practitioners trained at the McTimoney Chiropractic School, Oxford, who use the initials CP or MIPC.)

The College of Osteopaths Practitioners' Association,
21 Manor Road North,
Wallington,
Surrey SM6 7NS
Tel. 081 398 3308
(For register of graduates from the College of Osteopaths, using the initials FCO or MCO.)

The General Council and Register of Osteopaths,
56 London Street,
Reading,
Berks RG1 4SQ
Tel. 0734 576 585

For register of practitioners trained at:
  The British School of Osteopathy,
  1-4 Suffolk Street,
  London SW17 4HG
  Tel. 071 839 2060
  (Who use the initials DO, MRO.)

  The British School of Naturopathy and Osteopathy,
  6 Netherhall Gardens,
  London NW3 5RR
  Tel. 071 435 8728
  (They use the initials DO, MRO.)

  The European School of Osteopathy,
  104 Tonbridge Road,
  Maidstone,
  Kent ME16 8SL
  Tel. 0622 671558
  (They use the initials DO, MRO.)

The London School of Osteopathy,
Registered office: 110 Lower Richmond Road,
Putney,
London SW15 1LN
Tel. 081 785 2267
(For register of graduates of the school, who are members of the Natural Therapeutic and Osteopathic Society and use the initials DO, MNTOS.)

Further Reading

Leon Chaitow, *Osteopathy*, (Thorsons, 1982)
Paul Masters, *Osteopathy for Everyone*, (Penguin, 1988)
Edward Triance, *Osteopathy: A Patient's Guide*, (Thorsons, 1986)

13. Reflexology and reflex zone therapy

'In the vast majority of the people I treat,' says a former nurse turned reflexologist, 'by the time I get to the second foot, their heads are nodding.' Reflexology is yet another complementary therapy that provides deep relaxation as well as therapeutic treatment for a number of ailments. Its origins are very old: an Ancient Egyptian wall painting shows two people having their feet treated. Reflexology was rediscovered in the 1920s by an American physician Dr William Fitzgerald, and is growing in popularity today.

Like acupuncture, it is based on the theory that there are channels of energy flowing through the body. These channels are not identical, yet both therapies are effective — which is one of those mysteries of alternative medicine. In the case of reflexology, there are ten channels, which can be tapped into through specific reflex zones in the feet and hands. The feet themselves represent a kind of map of the body, with the big toes relating to the head and neck, and the bony side of the foot to the spine; reflex points for the liver, kidneys and other organs are found in the soft part of the arch, and so on.

Reflexologists are trained to sense energy blockages in the feet, and massage techniques to unblock them, stimulating the energy flow, and encouraging the body to heal itself. Some patients can actually sense the energy in the part of the body relating to the point on the foot being treated; it can feel like a mild electric shock.

You may be treated sitting up or lying down. The practitioner will give a complete treatment to both feet, and then focus on any problem areas. For insomnia, particular attention is likely to be given to the head area, including the pituitary gland (the master gland of the hormonal system) and to the adrenals, which may be overworked by stress. The solar plexus (about a third of the way down the sole of the foot) is another point that is likely to receive extra attention, and you may be asked to breathe deeply while it is being treated; this is excellent for stress.

Reflexology is particularly good for conditions involving congestion — sinusitis, migraine, asthma, a sluggish liver, fluid retention and so on. Sometimes people treated for such conditions experience a reaction as their bodies throw out toxins, possibly in the form of vomiting or diarrhoea, after which they feel very much better and clearer.

Reflexology is also good for releasing emotional congestion, especially when the therapist is receptive and a good counsellor. The reflexologist quoted in the first paragraph treated a woman who had been sleeping badly and feeling generally stressed since the recent death of her mother. During her mother's illness she had held back her emotions in order to be 'strong for the family'. After two treatments she found herself in floods of tears; the reflexologist reassured her that this was absolutely right and healthy: there had been an emotional build-up which needed to be released. The client understood the sense of this; following this episode she slept much better.

On the whole, treatment is fairly painless; now and again pressure on a particular site of trouble can hurt, but this does not last. Reflexology is in fact very good for the relief of chronic pain, possibly more effective than drugs and without the side effects. It is also helpful for hormonal imbalances and a variety of problems that may be affecting your sleep; after a treatment most people sleep extra well. As with other natural therapies, a course of several treatments will be needed to bring about a lasting effect, and patients can help themselves by following their practitioner's recommendations about diet and so on.

Reflex Zone Therapy, which works along very similar lines, is taught to and practised by qualified nurses and physiotherapists. Used in a maternity unit, it has been found particularly beneficial for post-birth problems, such as wind, and difficulty in passing urine. One new mother who was suffering from tension because of domestic problems asked for a sleeping tablet; since she needed to wake easily should her child need attention during the night, she was offered Reflex Zone Therapy instead. She was asleep before the treatment was complete, and woke six hours later to feed her baby.*

Finding a therapist

It is important to go to a well-trained practitioner; there are certain conditions (including the first three months of pregnancy and deep vein thrombosis) for which reflexology is contra-indicated.

There are a number of training schools. Names of practitioners in your locality can be obtained by writing, enclosing s.a.e., to:

*Margarita Evans, 'Reflex Zone Therapy for Mothers', *Nursing Times*, (24-30 January 1990)

The Institute for Complementary Medicine,
21 Portland Place,
London W1N 3AF
Tel. 071 636 9543

The British School of Reflex Zone Therapy of the Feet,
87 Oakington Avenue,
London HA9 8HY
Tel. 081 908 2201

Self-help

While it's not really feasible to treat one's own feet, you can learn from books to treat your hands, which contain a similar map of the body. Look out, too, for weekend or evening courses.

You can buy knobbly sandals claiming to give your feet a treatment while you walk around, but beware of wearing them for too long, which can over-stimulate the reflex zones and deplete your energy.

Further reading

Lucinda Lidell, *The Book of Massage*, (Ebury Press, 1984)
Hanne Marquardt, *Reflex Zone Therapy of the Feet*, (Thorsons, 1984)
Nicola Hall, *Reflexology: A Patient's Guide*, (Thorsons, 1986)

14. Shiatsu

Shiatsu, also called acupressure, is a form of oriental massage developed in Japan at the beginning of the twentieth century. It is based on the same principles as acupuncture, but uses the hands, fingers, knuckles and even elbows to stimulate the acupuncture points and rebalance the meridians. Practitioners also use the breath, breathing from the *hara*, the energy centre in the abdominal area, to direct energy into their hands.

Like acupuncture, Shiatsu helps to rebalance the body's energy system, relieving aches and pains, tension and stress. Ideally it is used to maintain health and vitality, rather than for curing disease, although in Japan, when practised by experienced practitioners, it can be as effective as acupuncture and medical herbalism.

Finding a practitioner

A list of therapists approved by the Professional Practitioners Association can be obtained from:

The Shiatsu Society,
Langside Park,
Kilbarchan,
Renfrewshire PA10 2EP
Tel. 05057 4657
(The national network for information on shiatsu.)

Self-help

A shiatsu practitioner may show you how to self-massage the points that will help you relax and improve your sleep. If you have someone to practise with, you can learn some self-help techniques from books, but if you have a medical condition, do not use it as a substitute for proper treatment. There is a form of self-shiatsu called Do-In; look out for evening classes or weekend workshops.

Further reading

Nigel Dawes and Fiona Harrold, *Massage Cures*, (Thorsons, 1990)
Lucinda Lidell, *The Book of Massage*, (Ebury Press, 1984)
Wataru Ohashi, *Do-it-yourself Shiatsu*, (Unwin paperbacks, 1979)

15. Spiritual healing

Spiritual healing, with its calming and uplifting effects on mind and body, can be extremely helpful with insomnia. It is also compatible with any other treatment you may be having, whether physical or psychological. Healing is numerically by far the largest of the natural therapies, with around 8,000 healer members in the Confederation of Healing Organizations, and probably as many outside it.

Some people are wary of healing because it is not fully explicable, and because of its supernatural associations. However, it is probably a perfectly natural human ability, which is beginning to come into its own. Today many doctors, as well as alternative practitioners, recognize that human beings consist of more than the visible, tangible physical body. Healing works primarily on the energy system, thus simultaneously treating mental, emotional and physical problems.

The Confederation of Healing Organizations, founded in the early 1980s, has done much to change the image of healers and make it more acceptable to the medical profession. The CHO is an umbrella organization for a number of different healing groups; although they have somewhat different philosophies and explanations for healing, its members are bound by a common code of conduct. The CHO aims to work in co-operation with the medical profession, and is conducting trials into the results of healing, supervised by medical experts. It has also encouraged the setting up of proper healer training courses.

Healers hold a variety of beliefs, and belong to all kinds of religious denominations, or none. There should be nothing weird about a healing session, provided you don't fall into the hands of a charlatan — unfortunately there are a few around. While many healers are spiritualists and regard their gifts as being assisted by spirit helpers, this is by no means always the case. These days, the power of healing is often explained in terms of the body's energy system, rather than in terms of spirits.

What is common to almost every healer is the belief in a cosmic or divine energy which is totally benign and loving. Healers see themselves as channels for this energy, which is transferred to patients through their hands (or by thought, in the case of distant healing). Imbalances caused by emotional trauma, and physical and nutritional stress, appear first within the energy field, before becoming consolidated in bodily symptoms. So it is in the energy field that healing starts. The transference of healing energy restores harmony to mind, body and spirit — hence the term 'spiritual healing'.

A healing session can last from 20 minutes to an hour. The

healer will usually chat with you first, and then ask you to sit or lie down; you don't have to remove any clothing. Many of them work almost purely in the energy field around the body, in which they can sense areas where there are problems. Others will lay their hands directly on painful areas, often relieving pain very rapidly. Many combine the two techniques.

Results are rarely instant or miraculous. The time it will take to bring about a cure or improvement depends very much on the condition of the individual patients and how long they have had their problem. Although faith is not necessary, patients can aid the healing process by being receptive and open minded. Some people feel the energy flowing from the healer as a hot or cold current, or a pleasant tingling. It is not necessary to feel anything, however, for healing to take effect.

Healing is usually a very relaxing experience; some people go to sleep during a session, and many sleep extra well afterwards. Patients often leave a session feeling emotionally and spiritually uplifted. Healers can also provide regular support for people going through difficult times, and help them to build up their own inner resources. Sometimes during a healing session patients find themselves crying, releasing pent-up stress or grief.

Many healers have clairvoyant or strongly intuitive gifts, which can help them to pinpoint the causes of people's problems. Many, too, are excellent intuitive counsellors, and healer training courses increasingly emphasize the development of counselling skills. It is important, they say, to heal not only the physical but the emotional/spiritual causes of illness. A number of them encourage patients to take part in the release of past stresses, through visualization, meditation, and forgiveness.

Some use aids like colour therapy (either projecting colour mentally, or using coloured lamps), gems and crystals, sound and even movement. Some call themselves 'etheric healers' or 'subtle energy healers'. And an increasing number of practitioners in other natural therapies also have healing gifts which can add a whole extra dimension to their treatment, whether or not they announce this fact. A number of these belong to the Association of Therapeutic Healers, listed below.

One woman began seeing a healer specifically for her insomnia, which had been extremely severe for several years; she was only sleeping for two or three hours a night. She had a number of emotional problems and, having decided to sort herself out, was also seeing a psychotherapist. Initially she found herself sleeping much better for two or three nights following each weekly healing session; as time went on, these two or three nights extended into seven nights a week.

Finding a healer

Many healers offer their services voluntarily or in exchange for donations; but as healing is becoming a therapeutic profession in its own right, a number now charge a standard fee (usually around £10-£20 but occasionally more.)

Beware of going to a healer about whom you know nothing, found through an advertisement. He or she may be absolutely on the level, but a few so-called healers do not work ethically.

The Confederation of Healing Organizations,
The Red and White House,
113 High Street,
Berkhamstead HP4 2DJ
Tel. 0442 870660
Its members include:

The Association of Therapeutic Healers,
Written enquiries to ATH c/o Celia Weller,
Derbyshire House,
Crank Road,
King's Moss,
St Helens,
Lancs WA11 8RJ
Telephone enquiries to Elizabeth St John, tel. 071 240 0176.
(Members combine healing gifts with other natural therapies —
kinesiology, counselling, massage, shiatsu, and so on)

The British Alliance of Healing Organizations,
c/o Mrs Pat Hissey,
26 Highfield Avenue,
Herne Bay CT6 6LM
Tel. 0227 373804

The Guild of Spiritualist Healers,
Guild House,
36 Newmarket,
Otley,
West Yorks LS21 3AE
Tel. 0943 462708

The National Federation of Spiritual Healers, NFSH,
Old Manor Farm Studio,
Church Street,
Sunbury-on-Thames,
Surrey TW16 6RG
Tel. 0932 83164/5
(The largest healing organization. Keeps a register of healer members, runs a number of healing clinics around the country)

Healing sections of the Spiritualists Association of Great Britain,
33 Belgrave Square,
London SW1X 8QL
Tel. 071 235 3351

Healing sections of the Spiritualists' National Union,
Redwoods,
Stanstead Hall,
Stansted Mountfichet,
Essex CM24 8UD
Tel. 0279 816363

The World Federation of Healing,
c/o Gilbert Anderson MNCP,
8a Devonshire Road,
Bexhill-on-Sea,
East Sussex TN40 1AS

Further reading

Anthea Courtenay, *Healing Now*, (Dent, 1991)
David Harvey, *The Power of Healing*, (Aquarian Press, 1983)
Eileen Herzberg, *Spiritual Healing: A Patient's Guide* (Thorsons 1988)
Philippa Pullar, *Spiritual and Lay Healing*, (Penguin Health 1988)
Allegra Taylor, *I Fly Out With Bright Feathers*, (Fontana, 1987)

Selective bibliography

Jo Douglas & Naomi Richman, *My Child Won't Sleep* (Penguin Books, 1984)

Jacob Empson, *Sleep and Dreaming* (Faber & Faber, 1989)

Peter Hauri, Ph.D, *The Sleep Disorders* (Upjohn, Michigan, 1977)

James Horne, *Why We Sleep: The Functions of Sleep in Humans and Other Mammals* (Oxford University Press, 1988)

Dr Peter Lambley, *Insomnia and Other Sleeping Problems: A Self-Help Guide to Sleep* (Sphere, 1982)

Stan Lindsay & Graham Powell (eds.), *A Handbook of Clinical Adult Psychology* (Gower, 1987)

Rosemary Nicol, *Sleep Like a Dream the Drug Free Way* (Sheldon Press, 1988)

Index